Essentially Raw

MARIE SARANTAKIS

Copyright © 2012 Marie Sarantakis.

All rights reserved.

ISBN: 0615615945
ISBN-13: 978-0615615943

A special thanks to Michael Skleney of BFD PhotoStudio for the back cover image, Ricardo Moura for the cover design of this publication, and Suzanne Hacker for the contributions obtained from her nutritional counsel.

DISCLAIMER

This book is not intended to help prevent, diagnose, or treat any physical condition(s). Do not attempt to medicate yourself of any ailments. It is imperative that you consult with your licensed healthcare provider. The author makes no implicit guarantees of the timeliness, accuracy, currency, or validity of any of the information provided. All of the recommendations rendered are opinions and should not constitute as legal and/or medical advice. The ideas expressed in this book are intended for general education purposes only. The author shall not be held liable of any damages, directly or indirectly, related to the applications or understandings of this publication.

This book is dedicated to Dr. Wayne Luther Thompson, my professor and mentor, who always encouraged me to follow my dreams.

CONTENTS

	Preface	i
1	Back to the Basics	1
2	You're So Vain	22
3	All About Alkalinity	32
4	The Art of Juicing	38
5	Fruit Guide	46
6	Vegetable Guide	61
7	The Rest of the Raw Pyramid	71
8	The Raw Carnivore	93
9	Ten Days Worth of Raw Recipes	106
10	Ten Takeaways for Success	136

FOREWORD *BY MITCHEL SCHWINDT, M.D.*

The statistics clearly support a disturbing trend in our society. The rise of obesity and the diseases associated with being overweight are rising at an alarming rate. This sad state of affairs is quite evident everywhere one looks; the end result of the standard American diet is evident.

While many look to medicine for the easy answer, the reality is that the most powerful tool is right in the kitchen. The power of natural and whole foods has been well established in the medical literature. This book will guide you through ten critical concepts and empower you to harness the benefits of a healthier diet.

This incredible book written by Marie Sarantakis captures the realistic and simple approach to healthy eating. Readers will see the benefits of eating whole foods and its' ability to transform lives.

As a physician, I see the ravages of unhealthy eating on a daily basis. The corollary is that through diet modification, incorporating whole and raw foods, such as fruits and vegetables, many patients are able to substantially improve their health. Common problems such as high blood pressure, elevated cholesterol and some forms of diabetes can be eliminated. Marie has done a superb job of enlightening her readers with an entertaining and enjoyable writing style.

Following the ten main points in Marie's book will allow readers to map out a plan for success. She shares a wealth of information in an easy to use format that is sure to transform the lives and health for those who apply this new knowledge.

Mitchel Schwindt, M.D. received his Emergency Medicine training at Butterworth Hospital (now Spectrum Health Campus as part of Michigan State). While there he served as chief resident and resident coordinator for the flight program. Dr. Schwindt currently practices in a variety of clinical settings, active in both clinical and non-clinical consulting roles. He serves as program director for a trauma program and provides medical direction and oversight in that role.

PREFACE

Growing up in a traditional Greek family we tended to eat fairly healthy. The Mediterranean Diet is acclaimed by many to be a cornerstone in promoting longevity and anti-aging. We ate a diet rich in healthy fats and a variety of freshly grown vegetables. It wasn't until elementary school that I had even heard of things such as Lunchables and Chef Boyardee. These were the favorites of the kids who mocked my horta (dandelion greens) and dolmadthes (stuffed grape leaves). But it wasn't all tomato and cucumber salads drenched in virgin olive oil. Like most Greeks, meat, bread, and potatoes were a staple in our household. Everything was drenched in a stick of butter.

I never questioned the foods I ate. I thought that our diet was pretty "normal" and even healthy. After all, the most artificial thing I would see used in our meals was a bouillon cube, and even that was taboo and unspoken. As I grew older I saw my loved ones develop high cholesterol and struggle with slight muffin tops (that were always blamed on water retention of course). Watching them pop pills and skip meals I started to think, there must be a better way.

I became intrigued with juicing. That quickly turned into an appreciation for organic foods. Slowly I started to have less of a craving for meat and carbs but rather yearn for flavorful grown foods that were nutritional powerhouses. It's a natural progression; the better you eat, the harder it is to ever go back to facing that artificially colored yellow nacho cheese. It won't even seem remotely appealing to you.

That is the point of this book, to increase the amount of good food in your diet. You do not need to make some radical conversion into the raw lifestyle. It's not some weird new age cult that you have to extradite yourself from the normal world in order to belong. It's simply about integrating more fresh, uncooked food into your diet. It's not all or nothing, but it is necessary to start making wiser meal choices in a society where it's so easy to go wrong. Basically, we all must go *Essentially Raw*.

1 BACK TO THE BASICS

In a society with so many options and the constant inundation of new information we can become overwhelmed and confused when defining "healthy eating". We get hung up on new fad diets, while tossing them by the wayside for that new greasy special advertised on the evening commute. Before we know it, we find ourselves yet again at a drive-thru window. Eating healthy is simple. It's about going back to the basics. Forget about obsessing over your gluten-free pizza crust and start looking at your diet as a whole. I cannot get over how many times I hear people commending themselves over eating baked potato chips, and honestly believing that they are doing their body good. No, you are not doing your body some sort of favor, simply you are doing it less harm.

My other pet-peeve... pretzels. All over corporate America I hear reformed fast-food junkies patting themselves on the back over eating a Ziploc baggie of pretzels. I'm not saying that pretzels are bad for one's health, but all too often people are misinformed and believe that they are putting a superfood into their body. Perhaps in relation to a candy bar, then yes. Just because something is better for you, doesn't mean it's good for you. For example, french fries made with sea salt are to some slight degree better for you than those made with regular salt. They are not, however, something that is good for you. You should not be consuming mounds of sea salt covered pretzels or fries in the name of nutrition.

Healthy is often defined by what we are led to believe by marketing gurus. I partially blame advertisers for tempting consumers into misinformation, but I mostly blame the consumers themselves for buying into propaganda without wanting to become more informed in their food choices. There are some other notorious masked offenders out there parading around cloaked in costumes of nutrition, such as yogurt and protein bars. Yogurt can be wonderful, especially the Greek versions, but the majority of what is lining your grocery store's shelves is loaded with more sugar than a bakery good. Opt for plain yogurt whenever possible. Sweeten it yourself with some fresh berries or honey. Another devil is disguise may be the protein bar. Be cautious, you might be eating something that is similar in calories and sugar to a brownie. And that doesn't really taste as good as one. Simply, read your labels. Or even better yet, eliminate labels from your diet as much as possible.

There's a really easy method to doing just that. When you go to the grocery store, shop the perimeter of the store. The more you can ignore all of the junk in the center aisles, the better. Such a simple concept and so incredibly beneficial. I'm not really a nutritionist, rather a "common-sensist". I suggest that you learn as much as you can and then employ that knowledge into action with your food choices. Avoid that which is bad for you and eat more of that which is good for you. Sounds simple, doesn't it? Even though we often intuitively distinguish the good options from the bad, more often than not, we still opt for bad food. Life is too short not to eat well, and it's even shorter if we don't.

I know what you're thinking. Does the food I eat really make that huge of an impact on my health? You bet it does! Think of it this way. When you consume one little Advil at the onset of a headache, you experience relief. That pill doesn't miraculously know where to go and target only the region ailing you. Rather that pill has an effect on a molecular level, affecting every cell in your body. If something so tiny can contribute to how every cell in your body feels, imagine what an entire meal is capable of.

Let us use another analogy. Pretend you have a brand new shiny Mercedes SLK. You buy it new, and it's in pristine condition. It's been nurtured mechanically. You find out that the car is specifically manufactured to run on a premium octane gas. But you notice that everyone else is using regular. Gas prices are high so you decide to cut corners and fill it up with regular gasoline too. After all, what can it hurt? Everybody else is doing it. You are enjoying your savings and not really all too concerned about the long-term consequences. Immediately you start to notice it's not running optimally. The car starts hesitating and almost seems as though it is slowly choking. The power is simply lacking. It's not a huge deal, so you just keep on doing it, thinking it's still a worthwhile cut. Then down the road you start having some major problems with the fuel system. You become faced with the reality that your decisions weren't all that prudent.

Unfortunately people are doing the very same thing with their bodies. Generally speaking we are born in a healthy condition. Our bodies have not yet been tarnished by Poptarts and chimichangas. We start ingesting sugary cereals and giant sodas thinking that everybody else is doing it, so it's normal. They're okay. So, we keep on doing it. We lack energy, but don't question it all too much. What does it matter? Isn't the payoff of ordering off the Dollar Menu a decent tradeoff for a little less energy? You may think I'll start eating better, eventually when I have the time and can afford it. Pretty soon your body adjusts and becomes used to eating the junk. Then as you start to age that's when the trouble starts. Your organs have not been well taken care of. You are more susceptible for all sorts of major health issues. If you are not providing your car or your body the fuel which it needs, you are going to suffer as a result in exchange for only some short term gains. The Standard American Diet has such an appropriate acronym, SAD. And that is exactly what it is.

The more processed foods we can replace with their fresh alternatives, the better off we will be. We will look and feel so much better. It's silly to keep feeding our bodies poison and not expect any ramifications. One of the greatest ways to start eating in a manner that pleases your body is to start eating more raw foods. The raw diet is rich in enzymes, amino acids, and vitamins while low in calories, fat, and sugar.

Here are some frequently asked questions that will address the common concerns associated with going raw...

First and Foremost, **What is The Raw Diet?**

Exactly what it sounds like...eating uncooked foods. This usually includes foods cooked under 120 degrees Fahrenheit. You can even heat many soups and casseroles up to this temperature, and they still preserve nutrients that would have been lost at higher temperatures. You will find this 120 degree number to be a ballpark figure, within a range of ten degrees, depending on the raw food guide that you are reading. The important thing to remember is that when you heat foods above 130 degrees Fahrenheit you will be destroying many of the micronutrients, enzymes, and amino acids that are readily available. A popular misconception is that you will be eating all cold foods. That's far from true. You can heat up foods to a certain extent, while also replicating the texture of cooked foods through dehydration.

In general the foods you will most often enjoy on the raw food diet are fruits, vegetables, seaweed, spouts, herbs, nuts, seeds, and possibly sashimi. Add and eliminate at your will. Most will eliminate meat and animal products. However there are some raw meat eaters out there, but they are a minority. Proceed with raw meats at your own risk. We will discuss this in further detail a little later. Some will also eliminate cooked grains from their diets. While others also give up dairy and anything that has been pasteurized, such as canned foods.

Pasteurization: *The process of heating a liquid to destroy protozoa, mold, bacteria, and yeast.*

You certainly don't have to give up all or any of that though. Many still eat cooked fish, and even chicken. The most important thing I suggest about taking on the raw diet, is that you need to make it your own. Your preferences, needs, and body are unique. Do what feels right. I want to provide you with all of the information possible to help you best decide what it is that you want to eliminate and incorporate into your diet. The main objective is that you begin eat more foods raw than ever before.

Unlike you do with most diets, when eating raw it's not really all that necessary to regulate the amount of food you eat. Fresh food is just not that high in calories, while easily capable of satisfying your body's nutritional demands. Certainly there are exceptions to this rule, but for the most part, eat until you are satisfied. Due to the high water content of the fruits and vegetables you are eating you will likely feel more steadily full rather than filled to the rim with your belt too tight as you do at Thanksgiving Dinner.

It's not so much about quantity, as it is about the quality of food you eat. We tend to overeat the junk because our bodies are still craving more nutrients. We may be stuffed to the gills, but our bodies are still asking for more because they are lacking the vital things they need. You want the raw foods that you consume to be as fresh and as unprocessed as they can be. Choose organic whenever possible.

Organic Food: *Food that has not been irradiated, covered with pesticides, filled with preservatives, nor been genetically modified.*

Genetically Modified Organism (GMOs): *Food created for human consumption using molecular biology to furnish the desired traits.*

Three different governmental agencies are responsible for overseeing GMO food safety.

The **Environmental Protection Agency (EPA)** is in charge of inspecting the production plants for environmental safety.

The **U.S. Department of Agriculture (USDA)** determines whether the food is safe for production.

The **Food and Drug Administration (FDA)** decides whether or not the resulting food is safe enough to eat.

Currently genetically modified foods do not have to identify themselves by federal law. You would not know the difference between a regular old tomato and one that has been genetically modified at the grocery store. There is a lot of pressure being pushed forward by consumer interest groups hoping to see these foods be required to display labels or some form of distinction in the near future. The FDA's current stance on the matter is that genetically modified foods are the equivalent to regular foods and do not impose any threat to the general public. Therefore they see no need to provide mandatory distinction to the consumer.

Why should I eat organic foods?

The pesticides, herbicides, fertilizers, hormones, sewer sludge, antibiotics, and whatever else is contained in or on inorganic food can be toxic. You're putting a slow and cruel poison into your body that is not meant to be there. Natural foods are grown without the inundation of these harmful chemicals or irradiation. Not only do these foods taste better, they are better for you. Surprisingly they have a better flavor even without all these fillers. Plus, organic fruits and veggies can contain around a 40% higher level of antioxidants, than their non-organic counterparts. When a plant grows in nature it releases antioxidants to protect itself from insects and other plants. When modified it does not need to develop these antioxidants since a pesticide is performing that task instead. Increased antioxidants mean better protection against certain cancers.

Studies in rats have shown that those who ate organically grown food were slimmer, slept better, and had greater immunity. Does it mean the same is true for humans? Well it's not certain, but I think we can make a pretty good inference.

Buyer Beware: A lot of products emulate being organic by stating that they are "natural". These food products are not necessarily "organic". They are often times genetically modified and deceive undiscerning consumers.

Meat can also be organic. According to USDA standards organically raised animals must be free to move around, allowed outdoors, experience direct sunlight, breathe fresh air, and be provided with "dry" bedding. Regular livestock is often pumped with hormones (to grow faster), fed grotesque meals of by-products, and raised in cages where the animal is confined in its own filth, often without even enough room to ever lay down. Since these animals are raised in mass quantities and are in such close proximity, disease can become rampant. Antibiotics are used to prevent the spread of disease, but as a result you are eating these medications in your meat as well. It's no wonder humans are becoming more resistant to antibiotics. With organic meat, antibiotics are only given to animals that are actually sick, not as a routine preventative procedure. Not only are organic, grass-fed meats missing all of these harmful things, they contain more vitamins C/E, Omega-3s, and beta carotene.

If I choose to go on a Raw Diet do I NEED to go organic?

"Need" is a strong word. Simply put, no, you do not. But you should strongly consider it. Why are you going raw in the first place? If the reason is for health, then it just makes sense to go organic. Plus, it tastes so much better. Who doesn't want scrumptious food? Yes, it can be more costly and more challenging to find, but well worth your efforts. Rinsing off regular produce in the kitchen sink gets rid of some of the surface residues, but will not eliminate that which has been absorbed within.

Keep in mind organic fruits and vegetables tend to be smaller than their counterparts. Do not let the small size fool you though, they contain way more flavor.

Is it hard to make the switch?

A little, but it's probably easier than you think. It's critical to have realistic expectations. Going raw is not something that has to be all or nothing. You don't have to give up all of your favorite treats at once, or even ever. The more healthful food you begin to eat, the more you start to crave it. The cells in our taste buds regenerate every ten to fourteen days. Think of it this way, each time they do, it is a new opportunity to retrain your cravings.

Just as with exercising or starting any new sort of regiment, it's best to begin with a family member or friend. If you are going through the experience with someone else, not only will some of the practical challenges be eliminated, but it will be more fun. You can have a blast learning together and experimenting with new dishes.

What do I need in order to get started?

Your kitchen should be equipped with a blender, juicer, some sort of steamer, and food processor. If you're really serious about going raw, also purchase a dehydrator. It's what us raw foodies use instead of an oven. A dehydrator will enable you to replicate the texture of some of your favorite cooked meals, while keeping them in their raw form. However, a lot of recipes that call for a dehydrator can be quite time consuming. Plan ahead. A trip to your local health food store wouldn't hurt either. In addition to these tools, you will also need to maintain patience and exercise your will power.

Does eating raw mean that I have to give up desserts?

Absolutely not! It just means going guilt free. Even those who are 100% raw can still enjoy their fair share of sweets. Raw agave nectar is actually a common sweetener that replaces white refined, granulated sugar. Stevia is another favorite taking over the raw world. A dehydrator will enable you to create things like pie crusts and cookies. Best of all, you can't burn them. You can even still enjoy chocolate cake, made with cocoa powder, nuts, and dates. There are all sorts of raw frosting recipes and even truffles. If you're not opposed to using animal products you can still enjoy honey as a sweetener. Another less common option is dried cane sugar. Don't forget the healthiest option of all, you can utilize fruits (especially dates) to add a natural sweetness to many dishes.

Isn't going raw incredibly expensive?

Just as with any type of food shopping, it's all about your preferences. It certainly can be, but that goes for just about any meal plan. Organic food does tend to be more expensive, but it is of a higher quality. Yes, shopping at Whole Foods will be pricier than getting all of your groceries from Wal-Mart. You can stay raw and frugal, but to do so you have to become an informed shopper for your local area. One way to keep prices down is to know what fruits are in season when and to take a peek down your frozen foods aisle. There are certain fruits and veggies that you want to ensure that you buy organic due to their pesticide levels. Then there are others that you can purchase through more conventional means. Generally speaking foods with thinner skins should be purchased organically.

I like to obey the following rules....

Always Buy Organic: Apples, Celery, Grapes, Peaches, Pears, Potatoes, Spinach, and Strawberries

Okay to Buy Regular: Asparagus, Avocados, Bananas, Broccoli, Mangos, and Onions

As with all of the products you purchase for your home, check out your options to buy in bulk and also the price of purchasing from specialty food stores online. Rather than loading up on calorie fillers from your local Dollar Menu you may have to work a little harder to find a more nutritious raw alternative. I'm not going to lie to you and tell you that it's always easy, but I will say that it is well worth your effort.

What do you call somebody who eats primarily raw?

There are quite a few terms out there. Some of the most common are raw-foodist, living-foodist, and rawist. We will use these terms interchangeably. Your friends may refer to you as crazy, weirdo, a nut, etc. Don't worry, you'll live longer and get the last laugh.

Do rawists eat meat?

Some do, some don't. It's up to you really. There are several types of rawists out there. Here are a few of the different sub-categories.

Vegan - A vegan does not eat anything that comes from an animal, such as flesh (meat, poultry and seafood) or animal products (eggs and dairy). They often do not wear any clothing made of animals (i.e., leather, silk, wool, etc.). Some vegans also exclude yeast products and honey from their diets. How strict one chooses to go vegan greatly varies. The typical diet of a raw vegan consists of fruits, vegetables, nuts, seeds and sprouted grains and legumes.

Among raw vegans there are even more limited diets such as...

Juicearians - Just like the name suggests, a juiceraian mainly lives on juiced foods. They believe it's an excellent method to cleanse the body and possess a great deal more energy. They don't live off of store bought juices, rather have a juicer at home and juice the fruits and vegetables that they enjoy to create their meals. Juicing enables the body to process the vitamins and minerals quickly and efficiently. We will discuss juicing in depth in a later chapter.

Fruitarians - Yeah, you guessed it...these guys eat a diet composed mainly of fruit (generally speaking 75% or more). This is a very restrictive diet and people have to be extremely careful to ensure that they are receiving enough protein and Vitamin B12 (in addition to many other necessary vitamins). Deficiencies are quite prevalent on this diet since it is so incredibly limited. Some people become fruitarians for spiritual reasons, as they do not want to kill anything, including plants. These folks are called *ahimsa fruitarians*. They may even only eat fruit that has already fallen and not pick it themselves. As you can imagine some people take it to such an extreme that it can lead to social isolation.

Did you know that Steve Jobs was a famous fruitarian for a period of time?

"I was actually a fruitarian at that point in time. I ate only fruit. Now I'm a garbage can like everyone else. And we were about three months late in filing a fictitious business name so I threatened to call the company Apple Computer unless someone suggested a more interesting name by five o'clock that day. Hoping to stimulate creativity. And it stuck. And that's why we're called Apple."

- **Steve Jobs**

Other famous fruitarians include Adam and Eve (remember the apple) and Leonardo DaVinci. Even Gandhi was a semi-fruitarian.

If you think eating only fruit is limited, how about this one...

Sproutarians- Sproutarians eat a diet mainly consisting of sprouts (alfalfa, peas, fennel, etc.). You can sprout just about any raw seed. Sprouts are incredibly nutritious since they contain protein, carbohydrates, and oils. During the germination of a seed, there is the development of natural sugars and predigested amino acids that the plant processes as food. Sprouts are extremely healthy since they contain the life force within them that has the ability of generating cells. Due to this cellular regeneration ability, sprouts are thought to be a food that can slow down the aging processes in the human body. They also contain an extremely high vitamin content.

If you find these options a little extreme, but want to eliminated or greatly decrease your animal consumption then vegetarianism may be a good alternative. A vegetarian can be a vegan, but the rules that they follow are a little less strict. A raw vegetarian diet excludes meat, but often allows for dairy and eggs (and sometimes even fish). Vegetarian often implies one of the following categories:

Ovo Vegetarian – Similar to a vegan, but who also consumes eggs.

Lacto Vegetarian – Similar to a vegan, but who also consumes milk and cheese.

Ovo-Lacto Vegetarian – Similar to a vegan, but who also consumes eggs, cheese, and milk. (This is the most prevalent type of vegetarian.)

Pescetarian – Similar to a vegan, but who also eats fish.

Famous Pescetarians Include: *Howard Stern, Mary Tyler Moore, and Ted Danson.*

Then there is an even less common non-vegan and non-vegetarian raw group that actually does consume animals, and in their raw state. They follow the **Raw Meat Diet**. Be very cautious if going this route. I certainly don't advise it. Especially in today's world, our meat is so precarious. I have a profound respect for those who do it, but simply feel it's not worth the risk unless you really know the history of your meat. And even still, it's still risky territory. Uncooked, or even low-temperature cooked, meats can make you very ill since the temperature never reaches the point where it is able to kill the bacteria present. On this particular diet, meat is usually not cooked above the temperature of 104 degrees Fahrenheit.

A subtype of raw meat eaters are those who follow **The Primal Diet**. Basically you will be emulating the eating habits of a caveman. It consists of fatty meats, milk, honey, and minimal fruit, all of them raw. The founder of this diet is Aajonus Vonderplanitz who claims to have experienced a remarkable cure from cancer eating this way. It is estimated that he has somewhere around 20,000 followers in North America. His diet is controversial and intriguing. To learn more about Vonderplanitz you can read his books "The Recipe for Living Without Disease" and "We Want To Live".

Just how raw should I go?

A mistake I often see is that people go into a diet, for weight loss and/or health related reasons, with so much blind enthusiasm. They are committed wholeheartedly. In fact, they give up all of the guilty pleasures they once loved in favor of their new meal plan cold turkey. As a result, at a weak moment they cheat. Then they do it again and then once more. The next time that they cheat on their diet they consume as much junk as they can, so they can justify it as just this one time. Slowly they fall off the bandwagon. Dieting goes from a positive, to a penitentiary experience. Do not make this mistake. I recommend a slow integration of adding positive things in to your diet, so that eventually you start to crave the acquired taste of that which is good for you.

Going raw does not have to be all or nothing. In fact, I do not suggest that it should be. That is why I use the word "essentially" in the title. You want a plentiful amount of your diet to be raw, but not all. Plus, raw foods are necessary (aka; "essential") for optimal health. It's not however necessary to make a 100% conversion, but let's face it, most of us are extremely deficient in our fresh fruit and vegetable intake, and need to work at consuming more.

Extreme diets are unrealistic and for the most part they are ineffective. If you have been eating a varied diet for your entire life, it is not healthy to suddenly convert to anything drastically different. No need to shock your body, nor mind. Sudden dietary changes often lead to failure. You want to slowly acclimate into a new style of eating with your routine because it may very well be challenging to give up some of your old habits. Many people incorporate eating more raw foods into their diet while still enjoying their guilty pleasures...meat, cooked foods, and sweets of all sorts. Just how much you want to integrate raw foods into your diet and how quickly is completely up to you. You may choose to go completely vegan raw and be anxious to begin right away. If that's the type of person you are, this is your goal, and you have a track record of success becoming fully committed to something so quickly, then by all means, go all in. My aim here is not to stop you from eating cooked foods altogether, but to give you the most information possible so that you will be able to make a well-informed decision based on your needs. Hopefully you will find that your diet is improved as a result thereof. Going raw is just as much about what you have to unlearn, as what you learn. A raw diet will be much more successful if you consistently integrate raw foods as at least 51% of your meal plan, rather than going 100% for just a couple of weeks. I emphasize long term success, rather than temporary boosts that lead to falling off the wagon.

When we set ourselves up for such high expectations, especially unnecessarily, we can easily become discouraged. We start to cheat, and then it deteriorates from there until we feel as though we have failed. Do not set yourself up for failure. I know it's hard when you want to begin something new. You want to go all in. But I'm telling you, stay grounded and remain in it for the long-haul. Slow but steady wins the race. At first do not focus on what to take out of your diet but rather what to add into it. Slowly replace foods with their healthier counterparts and you will be less hungry for the junk. For example, I took my morning Starbucks latte and replaced it with a smoothie. Sure, I experienced caffeine withdrawals at first. But after a couple of days, I actually found that the energy I was enjoying out of my smoothie was just as potent as that of my sugary caffeinated coffee.

A lot of literature suggests that when going raw 75-100% of your diet should be uncooked. Just how raw you want to go may be something that you base on your motive. If you are converting for overall health, I suggest that making at least half of your diet raw is a wise choice. You can then choose to go up in your percentage over time. If you have a particular health ailment or are converting for the purpose of losing weight, you may want to go even higher in your percentage. Personally I advocate a goal ratio of around 51% for the average population, with one or two juices thrown in throughout the day. I add that extra little 1% to emphasize goal of making the majority of your diet raw. I believe that somewhere around half your consumption ratio is a little more realistic than what most raw food experts advocate. It's certainly an easier place to start. It won't take as much time or money as going completely raw, but you will reap some great benefits. For the average healthy person, this is sufficient.

If you are very dedicated and have the resources it's possible to go all in. But let's face it, the majority of us struggle having enough time, tenacity, and money to be able to live the raw lifestyle to its fullest (especially right off the bat, in the learning stage). And frankly, it may just be overkill. You don't want to unnecessarily struggle without the added benefits. If you begin going raw and amp up your raw levels as you go, you can then determine what ratio makes the most sense based on your lifestyle and dietary needs. If you are determined to go 100% raw, you really need to be careful to ensure that your diet is varied enough. While it can be incredibly empowering at first, you need to be careful that it won't be problematic in the long run. When making a dietary change this drastic you should always consult with your physician to confirm it's a good idea based on your medical history and needs.

Eating raw is not something that is one size fits all. There are no perfect meal plans, no proscribed percentages, nor magic foods. You have to eat what you enjoy and what makes your body feel good. The ironic thing is that currently the foods we run to for comfort in our daily lives are the very things that leave us feeling uncomfortable. A major part of hunger is emotional. Eating until you are stuffed isn't normal, eating until you are satiated is. You will notice when eating real and raw food your body will not feel exhausted after eating. In fact, you will feel energized.

What's wrong with cooking your food anyways?

Vitamins & Minerals are Destroyed – Depending on the temperature, cooking time, and method many of the precious vitamins and minerals naturally contained within your food can be destroyed. The extent of the loss is based on the aforementioned factors. While generally speaking cooking destroys some of the nutritional content, there are also exceptions to this rule. Certain things, like the lycopene of a tomato, can be best absorbed by the human body after having been cooked.

Enzymes are Killed - Enzymes are a critical part of digestion. Think of that bogged down feeling after consuming your Thanksgiving dinner. That's your body at work creating the enzymes it needs to process the food. Sure, your body can create its own enzymes, as it does when you eat cooked foods, but raw foods contain enzymes of their very own. The ones that your body creates are not as efficient as those that are already within the food itself. As a result, they don't work as well, and the food may not be broken down as well as it could be. This leftover food can stick and rot in your intestinal wall, leaving a nice little breeding ground for parasites. (Caution: Sounds a lot scarier than it is. Eating cooked foods will not kill you nor cause an infestation of centipede-like-worm creatures to flourish in your body.) If all that doesn't scare you, maybe I can appeal to your vanity. Enzyme creation is associated with premature aging.

Life Force Energy is Removed - Live food contains a life energy that will in turn give your body energy. Someone once put it this way to me. A raw seed will grow in the soil, while a cooked seed will not. Think of it the same way with the things you put into your body. When you pick a fresh piece of fruit it will continue to ripen on its own for quite a while, however when you cook it, it stops ripening and quickly decays in to an unappetizing state. If you keep putting dead things into your body, you start looking like that limp and lifeless carcass yourself. Put live foods into your body and let their vibrant nourishment flourish within.

pH Factor is Altered - Cooking foods often raises their acidity level, and acidity is related to all sorts of diseases. Our goal is to keep our bodies slightly alkaline to not create a conducive environment for disease to flourish. Most organic raw foods do just that and can even help your body rid itself of excess acidity.

If the raw food diet is so incredible, why aren't more people doing it?

There are a plethora of reasons apathy, preference, price, knowledge, etc. Ordering a pizza on your smartphone for delivery takes just a few seconds, whereas grocery shopping and meal preparation are much more time consuming. People simply don't eat fresh anymore. They would rather eat food right out of a box, than figure out how to create something delicious and healthy. It takes research on the front end and patience in practice.

It is in fact more expensive to eat raw, especially if you are new at it and/or choose to go organic. Fast-food can provide you with some satisfaction and cheap. Eating raw on a budget takes effort and meal preparation takes time. When you eat fresh food you will have to shop more often since things spoil, especially when you take preservatives out of the picture.

While the raw food movement has not yet blanketed the nation with the popularity of the Snuggie, it is pretty notorious amongst those who want to keep up their appearances. Hollywood has long known the beauty secrets of raw food. One celebrity who looks remarkable for their age is Demi Moore. She is a major advocate and you have to admit, the raw diet is working for her. Woody Harrelson is another huge proponent. Designer Donna Karen said that she struggled at shedding off some extra pounds but found that a raw rich diet did wonders. Some other celebrities who are said to be fans of the raw movement are Jason Mraz, Cher, Natalie Portman, Angela Basset, Sting, Margaret Cho, Brooke Burke, Susan Sarandon, Edward Norton, Alicia Silverstone, Pierce Brosnan, and Uma Thurman.

The popularity of the raw diet is not confined to the west coast, but is generating quite a buzz throughout the entire United States. Raw restaurants are popping up everywhere and flourishing. Raw recipe books are being released more than ever before and new gurus are born every day.

Mainstream society is now seeing the need to accommodate those on a raw diet. In fact, Lufthansa Airlines has recently added a raw meal option to their international flights. I accredit much of the new found popularity to its success. You simply cannot hide its effectiveness The obesity endemic in America has led people down the path of trying new means of losing weight. People are becoming open to the idea of finding new ways to eat and acknowledging that their current habits simply just aren't working. When people give the raw diet a chance, they start to look and feel better. If you keep your food alive, it will do the same for you.

In times past, this sort of raw and/or vegan lifestyle was not thinkable. We did not have access to the nutritional supplements and vast array of information, for a well-balanced diet, which we have today. Our ancestors had to cook food to eliminate bacteria and survive on meat for strength. Times are a little different now. It is possible to remain vegan and enjoy a wide variety of non-animal foods, while remaining completely nourished. Even if you don't intend on going all raw or all vegan, adding more fruits and vegetables to your diet will be beneficial. No one is going to argue against the statement that fruits and vegetables are good for you. This is common sense.

I hear of people trying all kinds of fad diets in the name of weight loss and/or health. The Tapeworm Diet, The Blood Type Diet, The

12-Day Grapefruit Diet, The Cookie Diet, etc. Yes, each one of those is real. These diets gain a lot of popularity and then diminish as people fail to see results. Stop with all of this nonsense. Go back to the basics. Eat more fruits and veggies and find them in their purest state possible. You don't have to cook or do anything complicated. Just eat. It's that simple. If you're skeptical all you have to do is try it. You will be amazed at how invigorated and energized you will feel in just a short period of time.

I feel just fine eating cooked food. Why should I adjust my diet to include a greater percentage of raw foods?

Often times people confuse not ill, for healthy. Healthy means a lot more than that. To me it means you are not on a path headed towards illness. It means that your immunity and energy levels are strong. A lifestyle of junk food is not going to make you keel over dead instantly, rather it will gradually gnaw away at your at your body. Considering the way most of us eat, it's almost shocking seeing that the human body holds up as well as it does. Lots of people switch to eating better when they become ill. Imagine the strength of using raw foods as a means of prevention.

For the most part, I don't believe that disease strikes us randomly. Sure there is a certain part of genetics that leave us susceptible to predisposed risks. But if we know what we are vulnerable to, all the more reason to focus on preventative measures. Much of disease is a result of the lives we've lived. If we've taken care of our bodies properly, we should all enjoy living to a ripe old age. Disease strikes where there is vulnerability. I think hardly any of us can attest to eating all the right foods, avoiding environmental toxins, and exercising the way we should.

I'm not saying that everyone who is suffering from an illness has done it to themselves. Someone may eaten right and exercised every day, but have been exposed to environmental pollutants that made him/her ill. Or someone who has eaten raw, ensured they were getting all of the right nutrients, and was physically fit, may have eaten foods unknowingly filled with carcinogens. What I want to get across here is that there is that disease is usually a result of our life stories. It's the bad things that get in the way of our lives that cause disease, so why aren't we taking every precaution to ensure we live the healthiest lives possible? It may be impossible to prevent disease altogether, but let's feed our bodies with whatever promotes optimal health.

When it comes to healing I don't believe in simply suppressing symptoms, as is the main concern in modern medicine. We go to the doctor after something is wrong, not to stay healthy. We need to do everything we can to maintain health, not just regain it. Based on my research and personal experience, I feel that a diet that is rich in raw foods can help make that possible.

What should I be concerned about when going raw?

You need to ensure that you are nourishing your body adequately when eliminating certain things from your diet. The four things you want to be most concerned about are getting enough of are protein, vitamin B12, calcium, and iron. Protein, while notoriously found in animal products, is easy to obtain through nuts, seaweed, sprouts, leafy greens, and even certain fruits. It is necessary to build muscle. That's why it's such a staple for body builders. In addition, protein strengthens our immune system, maintains healthy brain function, and promotes cellular regeneration.

When going raw you should seriously consider taking a vitamin B12 supplement. B12 is critical in cell division and blood formation. Its deficiency can cause serious problems such as permanent nerve damage and severe anemia. In fact, it may be the number one thing that concerns people about going raw. Because of the gravity of its deficiency, I advocate integrating healthy small portions of meat and/or fish into your diet regularly. I am not a complete rawist, nor vegan, but completely understand those who are for ethical reasons. But in terms of health, a little meat will do you more good than harm. However if you want to remain vegan, you have to do your homework. Some sources of vitamin B12 include miso and seaweed, although they are certainly not reliable. Things grown in soil with traces of manure are also shown to have minimal amounts of B12. But once again... very, very little. Nutritional yeast, supplements, and B12 fortified foods (such as cereals) are the most reliable sources chosen by prudent vegans.

When it comes to calcium, rawists who are lacto and ovo-lacto vegetarians will not to be overly concerned since dairy is part of their normal diet. Unlike B12, calcium is an easier find for those who choose to be animal-free. They can obtain a healthy amount by incorporating enough tofu, leafy greens, and nuts into their diets. In addition, there are always calcium-fortified foods and even supplements to help fill in the gaps.

When you're not consuming red meat you have to be very careful not to become anemic. Anemia is actually so prevalent today, amongst the population at large, that it is considered to be the most common nutritional deficiency. To avoid this issue as a vegan you should enjoy regular servings of quinoa, spirulina, lentils, prune juice, and pumpkin seeds. Unfortunately consuming iron rich foods is not enough. You need to help your body process this iron into a usable form. To increase absorption, accompany the intake of iron with vitamin C and don't consume calcium within the same hour. The polyphenols in coffee can also hinder iron absorption.

In general, to help prevent becoming nutritionally deficient take a daily multi-vitamin. Deficiency is something we all have to worry about, not just those of us going raw. Whether you're a rawist, vegan, or strict chicken nugget eater, a multi-vitamin will do you good.

While many are concerned that eating raw will lead to a nutritional deficiency, the result is most often quite opposite. It's those living on cooked, processed food who are lacking a well rounded diet. Usually going raw will make you even more aware of what you are putting into your body and you will be less likely to lack the things which you need. If you're not feeling quite right, think about what you may be missing. Your body will tell you when something is wrong. Listen to it. Once again, we're resorting to common sense. Know what you need and be sure you are getting enough of it.

Is it true that eating raw is good for the environment?

Absolutely! "Going green" is one of those double entendres. Eat more greens and the planet benefits. If living longer and looking better don't motivate you then maybe reducing your carbon footprint will.

A world-wide vegetarian diet would greatly reduce the world's C02 emission. Assembly-line meat factories emit a substantial amount of greenhouse gases, pollute our water supply, and require incredible amounts of energy. If every person cut back eating meat just one day they would save enough grains to feed our entire world population a meal.

Since most rawists tend to go organic, they avoid eating foods that are drenched with the "Icky Ides" (herbicides, pesticides, etc.) All of these awful chemicals are not just limited to area where they are distributed, but spread across the entire planet in the water and food cycles. No living being is immune from all of the junk in the ground. The truth remains that we don't know the long term ramifications of the contaminants all around us.

Let us not forget, rain forests are destroyed to make room for the grains which are used to feed animals that are for slaughter. It is estimated that it takes approximately sixty pounds of animal feed to equal one pound of beef. Not only are these rain forests destroyed and the animals slaughtered, but all of that animal feed is soaked in a vast amount of chemicals and is genetically modified. Guess what... that nasty stuff still remains in the earth and is even more of it is directly injected into your body when you consume many meats. A majority of those who go raw are vegan, and of those who aren't, they hardly eat much meat in comparison to their Standard American Diet counterparts.

Final Words

While it can be challenging at first to become accustomed to eating raw, it can also be fun! It's not just about eating celery sticks. You get to learn new recipes and orient yourself with looking at foods in a totally new way. Once you have the basics down, you will start being able to replicate all of your favorite cooked foods in their raw form. If you keep a wide variety of fruits, veggies, and sprouts on hand it's easy to toss together an interesting salad quite simply. Besides, you wouldn't believe how many different types of fruits and vegetables there are that you've never even seen or heard of. Keep it simple at first; otherwise you will quickly be discouraged. It's easy to get caught up in a ten hour dehydrating project and frustrated. Most importantly, have realistic expectations. You won't convert your diet, lose weight, feel/look better overnight.

This new style of eating may pose some challenges until you get acclimated. Make sure you are integrating enough calcium and iron in to your diet. Meat and milk are the most common sources, but certainly not the only ones. You can absorb a ton of calcium, while staying raw and vegan, through sesame seeds. Let's not forget kale, prunes, seaweeds, leafy greens, and almonds. Iron is found in many of these same foods as well as beets, apricots, raisins, watermelon, flax seeds, pumpkin seeds, and sun-dried tomatoes. Find a way to integrate vitamin B12 into your meal plans, since it is vital to your wellbeing. And finally don't forget to remain aware of your protein intake.

Many people realize that a raw diet is going to help them improve their overall long-term health, but frankly this is often not enough of a reason to adjust their eating habits on a daily basis. Something I like to encourage people to do is to keep their sights on the superficial short-term benefits. You will start looking better rather quickly. It's amazing the ways we change our behavior for the sake of our looks, rather than for the sake of our health. Enjoy a nice serving of carrots and plums, and your skin's hue will thank you for it.

2 YOU'RE SO VAIN: THE BENEFITS OF GOING RAW

Beauty and health contribute to one another as cause and effect. They constantly work in tandem. A person who is perceived as beautiful is one who is healthy. Our conceptions of attractiveness lay based on what is considered healthy in a particular culture at a particular time. For the past several years tanning has spiked in popularity. I hardly attribute this fad having anything to do with Jersey Shore. Rather the appearance of a healthy glow symbolizes an active outdoor lifestyle and is symbolic of leisure time. Let's think about who is tanning. It's certainly not someone who is not cooped up indoors in a stressful work environment day in and day out. Generally it's someone who has enough time and money to relax in a tanning bad or casually sit along the beach. It seems like all affluent men and women, especially those on television, are dawning a dewy bronze glow. It's a sign of health and vitality. A life not burdened by stress. In centuries past a tan signified quite the opposite about a person. It meant you were working class, stuck outside in the blistering son, and a victim of a rough life. In those days fair skin was a sign of beauty. Beauty is always related to that which is healthy, but what is symbolic of health changes with place and time.

Another interesting variable regarding attractiveness and health is weight. In the mid-nineteenth century heavy set women were considered more attractive than those who were thin. Weight signified that a woman was healthy, fertile, and prosperous. In many cultures even today, this still reigns true. Although now in the United States obesity is an endemic. Drive-thru dinners are the norm and the reason that so many westerners are overweight is due to their poor lifestyle choices. The mainstream food that is readily available to us is typically garbage. Even in a grocery store, most of what you see in people's shopping carts is junk. You have to pretty much go to a health food store or organic grocery store to buy the food that would have been considered of an average quality in our grandparent's generation.

Nowadays a bigger-sized lady is inferred to have consumed large quantities of poor quality food and/or lacks the motivation to exercise. This harmful food and inactivity is inextricably linked to weight gain and in turn a ceaseless list of health problems. In modern society, a fit and lean body is symbolic of health, discipline, and vitality. Just as with the tanning scenario, it means that one is not constantly confined to a desk chair of a toxic work environment downing aspartame loaded sodas. It is assumed to be someone who has the time and energy to live an active life of leisure, while eating quality foods in small portions. Keep in mind weight is not a static judge of beauty, but a variable whose meaning is constantly in flux.

The only thing that is a constant in what is considered beautiful in all societies across all time is that health is always attractive. Reducing stress, getting adequate amounts of sleep, and exercise all positively contribute to our overall health, but one of the greatest factors of which we have control over is our diet. If you look better, you feel better... and if you feel better, you look better. Focus on health, and beauty will naturally flourish.

It amazes me how much time, money, and pain people endure to look good. Not that I am against looking hot.. I'm all about it!! All I'm saying is that it is so much easier to treat ourselves inside-out. It seems like people are so readily willing to drop a small fortune on a miracle skin cream or poisonous freezing injections rather than eat well and pop a vitamin. Think about it. Why aren't you replacing your fried chicken fingers for a plate of veggies? What good reason do you have not to take a vitamin? I can readily list you a hundred benefits, but not a single adverse affect. It starts with something that simple. One step at a time you can alter your lifestyle.

Now let's not misconstrue what we are dealing with here. Taking a Flintstone gummy vitamin and/or drinking a glass of fresh squeezed orange juice is not going to reverse your crow's feet, but years of taking care of your body properly will ensure that you do not prematurely age. Preventative maintenance is so much better than dealing with issues after they occur. I'm not saying that by eating raw and you will undergo a magical transformation and instantly attain beauty, but you can enhance your natural beauty so that you are living up to your full-potential. Seriously, the Big Mac is not doing you any favors.

Vanity is a virtue, a perfect impetus for change. Channel it properly and you will be looking amazing sooner than you can even imagine. The raw diet is notorious for its beauty benefits. Stop trying to camouflage your imperfect assets and discover your body's ability to heal itself. Here are some of the things you can expect by adhering to a mostly raw diet...

Reveal Youthful Skin - Our bodies are mostly composed of water. It only makes sense to replenish them with a clean water source, not sugary carbonated syrup. Fruits and veggies are a great host of pure hydration. Not only will your complexion improve, but your skin will appear hydrated. Dull, lackluster skin means that your body is experiencing deficiencies. When you eat the way nature intended, your body doesn't have to ration out the disbursement of its nutrients for survival, but instead can adequately furnish your entire body. The look and feel of our skin is a direct reflection of our inner conditions. Cutting out the saturated and trans fats from your diet will help clear up acne. Plus a nutrient rich diet will leave your skin looking fresh, young, and toned. All of the antioxidants contained within fruits and vegetables will help flush out the toxins that are in your system. Collagen, which keeps your skin looking plump and firm, is highly susceptible to free radical damage.

Maintain A Healthy Weight – When you eat the right food you feel full before you start packing on the calories that turn into a muffin top. Freshly grown foods are low in calories while high in fiber and water content. These types of foods will leave you feeling satiated, without packing on the pounds. Plus a diet rich in fruits and vegetables tends to be alkaline and help break down fatty acidic cells. And let's face it; it's hard to get fat by eating one too many carrots. Going raw is not a diet; it's a change in one's lifestyle. Your weight loss is going to be consistent and drastic if you convert to making a majority of your diet raw. The typical Western diet is loaded with sugars, fats, carbs, and processed garbage. Eliminate these things from your daily life and watch how the pounds will shed themselves. I really don't know of any diet out there that can ensure weight loss quite like going raw. It's practically effortless to lose weight once you go raw. Maintaining a healthy weight should not be for vanity alone, but for a variety of physical health-related reasons. Obesity contributes to the risk of heart disease, diabetes, high-cholesterol, and cancer.

Brighten Your Sclera - You can actually whiten the white part of your eyes naturally. I think all too often our eyes are one of the beauty elements that we overlook. Ironically so many people say what initially attracted them to their mate is that very feature. In the past I used to engage in quite a bit of commercial modeling. Sometimes I would sit along with the photographers and watch the editing process. The first thing the photographer would almost always do is whiten the teeth. Secondly, they would brighten the eyes. White sclera represent youth, health, and vitality. A poor diet makes them appear yellow and the small red blood vessels look inflamed.

Reverse Aging – Bring back the youth and vitality you once knew without all of the pain of plastic surgery and cost of expensive creams. I'm not saying that eating a cup of spirulina will substitute a facelift, but over time you will witness some noticeable improvements. Unlike Cher, you will be able to turn back time. Your skin will naturally glow and appear more plump. As a result of the increased hydration from your food sources, you will combat aging. Dry skin leads to wrinkles. Plus, the raw diet is rich in antioxidants which eliminate free radicals. When you give your body the nutrients it craves damaged cells can repair themselves. Cell regeneration will leave you looking and feeling more youthful. Berries and citrus can help promote collagen production while protecting your skin against sun damage. Foods that contain traces of sulfur, such as onions, red pepper, and garlic, will promote healthy skin, nails, and hair.

Possess More Energy – A vibrant personality is attractive. No one is drawn to a person who drags listlessly around tired and moping. Besides, when you have more energy you will be more active. You can get more done in a day and keep your body fit. Live foods have live energy. Your body does not have to work as hard in the digestion process and as a result that energy can be used elsewhere. Processed foods drain your body of energy while live foods will increase it. Raw food contains enzymes that are responsible for every chemical reaction that takes in your body. When your body has readily available enzymes you enhance its vitality.

Improve Your Mood - Guess what... when you look better, you feel better. All of the nasty stuff we put in our bodies, unsurprisingly makes us feel nasty. When you feel better you tend to be more active. When you do more, you burn more calories. The cycle of health consistently contributes upon itself.

Depression and mood swings are often rooted in nutritional deficiency. You know how when a small child is feeling tired or hungry they throw a tantrum. We really don't change that much as we grow older, we just learn to conceal it better. There are overwhelming numbers of personal accounts where people find years of depression start to vanish when going raw. This may be explained by improved self-image, increased health, boosted energy levels, among several other factors. While Americans are popping more pills for depression than ever before, holistic alternatives are finally starting to play a strong role in the arena of healing. Foods such as raw cacao, cauliflower, and whole grain oats are particularly effective at enhancing your mood.

Detoxify - All the healthy goodness of raw foods helps to push free radicals out of your system. Detoxification can reduce inflammation, enhance the look of your skin, and aid in weight loss. Even Oprah has dabbled in raw detoxification.

A raw food diet is not merely something done for superficial gain, but rather an incredible method for keeping your body in optimum health. I like to emphasize the beauty benefits because that's was most readily springs people into action. Here are some additional health benefits...

Promote Brain Health - Raw foods are known to improve your focus, concentration, and recall ability. Some claim it's a spiritual thing. When you are closer to the Source (with pure food from the Earth) you understand things more clearly. The more scientific explanation is that fresh foods help carry oxygen into your bloodstream. The chlorophyll of leafy greens and wheat grass are especially powerful in transporting oxygen to your brain.

Need Less Sleep - Crazy, I know. But it's a very common phenomenon reported by raw food eaters everywhere. Now don't get me wrong, get as much sleep as your body needs, but if you're body starts to need less sleep, don't be surprised. This is just another added bonus. Don't cut back on sleep intentionally after going raw, but see if your body naturally does so. I suppose there are a lot of rational explanations to this anomaly. Sleep is when the body repairs itself from the damage it has incurred, if you're not damaging your body, less healing is needed. Next, cooked food is difficult for the body to digest. Your body is not working as hard in the digestion process, leaving you with more energy. A raw diet also supports healthy insulin levels, which regulates your cortisol rhythm, that directly affects your sleep patterns. Finally when your body becomes less acidic, as it often does when going raw, research suggests that sleep and overall energy is improved. In summation, it is widely reported that your body will naturally wake up more alert and rested, and likely with even less sleep than ever before.

Stabilize Your Blood Sugar – We're all practically walking around in a sugar coma these days. Sweeteners are lurking in processed foods everywhere. When your blood sugar is in a healthy state, your mood is better. Think of a kid with too much sugar or not enough sleep... cranky. Well, the same is true of adults. We just sometimes shield it better.

Improve Fertility – When couples are experiencing infertility, depending on the reasoning, it is now becoming more often suggested by fertility experts that couples convert to a raw diet for a temporary period of time to see if they have any luck in conceiving naturally. Personally I think its junk food to blame, more than cooked food in general, for any link to infertility. If you go raw, you tend to eat healthier, and will fulfill more of your body's dietary needs.

Strengthen Your Immune System – I see people going through the trouble of getting a flu shot all of the time, yet if people took the time and energy to take care of their bodies properly, their immune systems would be capable of fighting off the common bug just fine on their very own. A diet that adequately provides enough nutrients and minerals goes a long way in keeping your body strong. In addition, it's important to get a sufficient amount of sleep, reduce stress, and stay active.

Prevent Diabetes – A raw diet does not in itself contain a lot of sugar. Sure there are the natural sugars found in fruits, but typically speaking you won't be consuming the loads of sugar that is packed hidden in most processed foods. High fructose corn syrup is lurking everywhere these days. The sugar found in fruit is much easier for your body to break down and digest. Studies show that a raw diet can even be quite effective in managing diabetes, but this should be done under the direction of a physician.

Ease Digestion – A 1930 clinical study by Dr. Paul Kouchakoff compared raw versus cooked diets, and their affect on the immune system. He discovered that in those eating primarily cooked foods that their white blood cell count would increase after eating. White blood cell count generally increases as a result of some sort of infection or exposure to a toxic chemical. What was extraordinary was that raw food did not have this same reaction when ingested. Sure your body can handle cooked food, that's fairly obvious. But the truth remains that raw food is less taxing for your body to breakdown. Raw foods are processed and excreted by the human body very easily.

Increase Life Expectancy – Eat the right foods, and God willing, you should expect to live a long healthy life. Raw foods can provide you with enzymes, phytochemicals, and natural hormones to promote longevity. Plus they will help keep you hydrated and your body adequately furnished with oxygen, which will slow premature aging and the decrease the likelihood of disease.

Stay Regular – A raw diet should provide you with more than an adequate amount of fiber to keep your bowel movements on track.

Increase Hydration – Way too many people are dehydrated these days and most don't even know it. You cannot get by on a day just drinking coffee and sodas. In fact, these things only dehydrate you further. Raw diets typically have a very high water content.

The Downsides Of Going Raw

While there are no major negative ramifications, you are at an increased risk of becoming nutritionally deficient when you start to remove things from your diet. But then again those who seem to be lacking the greatest amount of vital nutrients are those living on the Standard American Diet. Here are some of the potential downsides to going raw…

Flatulence - A lot of the foods that we eat on a raw diet can cause gas. Some examples of offenders include, but are not limited to, apples, pears, peaches, bananas, apricots, cauliflower, broccoli, carrots, corn, asparagus, artichokes, celery, and onions.

Detox Symptoms - As your body is eliminating all of the toxins that have accumulated from years of poor eating habits you may start to feel weak. Some people even experience flu-like symptoms. If you start feeling poorly, ensure that you are getting all of the nutrients that your body needs and transition your diet more slowly. Radical dietary transformations of any sort, good or bad, can leave you feeling unpleasant.

Snickers from Co-Workers & Friends - So what? If you eat right, you'll live longer than them anyways. We'll just see who gets the last laugh.

Feeling Hungry - It may take a while to re-learn just how much to eat. Make sure you eat until you feel full. Seems silly to say, but necessary nonetheless. Foods that lack nutritional value will fill you up fast, but leave you hungry soon after. Healthy food won't leave you feeling stuffed, but that's a good thing. You really don't want that weighed down, lazy feeling anyways. Healthy food will keep you feeling satisfied and energized.

Potential Weight Gain - Even though the result is, as expected, typically opposite, it has sometimes been reported that people gain weight. Instead of replacing bad food, with good food, they simply add more things to their diets. Eating a bunch of junk food and then adding a carrot juice and a side salad to your meal, is not going to result in you losing weight. You don't usually hear people saying they got a muffin top by eating too much broccoli, but I suppose it could happen if you dip it in enough ranch.

Practical Challenges - It takes more time and money to eat raw, especially at first. There is a lot of learning involved in the early stages. Besides, it's tempting to go for junk food when its so readily available. Are you going to go home and make a smoothie or are you going to just give in and stop by that drive-thru window? When you're out with family and friends at your local pizzeria, are you really going to opt for a salad or are you going to enjoy some of that cheesy greasy goodness? It's tough. That is exactly why I say you must be reasonable in your initial expectations. With time, raw food preparation becomes a breeze. You will soon find that is actually a lot easier than cooking with less cleanup time.

Vitamin Deficiencies - Although people with non-raw diets experience deficiencies all of the time, limiting the variety of foods you incorporate into your diet can come with a new set of challenges. Just be sure to take any necessary supplements and this problem is eliminated. Being conscious of your diet is crucial. People on a highly raw diet are susceptible of not getting enough iron, calcium, protein, or vitamin B12.

Boredom – This one is more of a misconception. Contrary to popular belief there are a ton of meal choices out there. You will not have to live on a diet of carrots like Bugs Bunny. You just have to relearn what's out there. I found that eating raw actually made food a lot more fun and exciting, but that took some time. You can pretty much replicate any cooked food favorite in its raw form.

Calculated Risk - Unpasteurized milk and uncooked fish/meat do contain an element of risk. You can choose whether you want to incorporate these foods into your diet in the safest manner possible or to not even deal with them whatsoever. By adding these foods into your diet you are less susceptible to deficiencies but at increased risk of foodborne illness. That is why I suggest that if you are not opposed to consuming meat for ethical reasons, you should try to incorporate some healthy serving sizes into your diet regularly. While this book is all about increasing the percentage of raw foods into your diet, animal products are one area that you should probably stick with high cooking temperatures. It is still incredibly easy to stay mostly raw while drinking pasteurized milk and consuming cooked meat.

Final Words

When you begin to compare the downsides of eating raw to the benefits, it seems no contest. Eating raw, wins by a landslide. You will start to look and feel better. Enhance your beauty and increase your lifespan, possibly even by decades. I cannot emphasize how much raw food will positively contribute to your overall lifestyle.

3 ALL ABOUT ALKALINITY

You're probably familiar with pH (potential hydrogen), but you've likely never taken it into consideration regarding your dietary needs. The pH scale ranges from 0 (extremely acidic) to 14 (extremely alkaline). Neutral lies smack dab in the center at 7. To put this into perspective, stomach acid is about a 1 and baking soda a 12. Water is the base measurement from which this scale is derived since it is fixed with the same amount of hydrogen ions (H+) and hydroxide ions (OH-). Something is considered alkaline when the OH- ions are greater than the number of H+, and acidic when the inverse is true. In order for something to grow well in soil its pH level has to be within a certain range. pH similarly needs to be balanced in a swimming pool or a fish tank. It's no surprise that the human body also needs to maintain a certain pH range in order to function properly. Optimally our blood should remain slightly alkaline, at around 7.365.

pH affects the body's ability to fight diseases and process nutrients. Bacteria and viruses thrive in acidic environments. Therefore our bodies remain slightly alkaline so that these harmful invaders cannot survive very easily. This type of environment allows the body to function sufficiently, while not being highly susceptible to disease. Alkalinity allows more oxygen to travel throughout the body, while acidity depletes it. You don't have to be that much more than a first grade scientist to know that oxygen is beneficial to the human body. When our body is not receiving an adequate supply of oxygen it is susceptible to cancers, heart disease, diabetes, as well as a plethora of other troubles.

While the importance of maintaining the proper pH balance is nothing new, it is gaining more attention than ever before because of how our diets have changed in recent decades. Americans are consuming more and more acidic foods, especially in everything that is processed. In order for the body to maintain slight alkalinity it has to work harder than ever and deprives itself of things such as calcium in the conversion process. This isn't dire nor tragic, as the body can compensate adequately on its own, but the question remains "at what cost". Do we want really want to unnecessarily be putting our bodies through this unneeded stress? Or does it even matter?

It's not that alkalinity is so much intrinsically better than acidity, but rather the Standard American Diet is so highly acidic. Our meals are loaded with red meat, soda, coffee, dairy, and refined sugars. Stress is yet another contributor of acid. An overindulgence in acidic foods and added stress will leave us feeling tired and prone to disease. In fact there's a term for this called acidosis. Acidosis has also been linked to bloating, heart burn, insomnia, brittle nails, irritability, weak teeth, fatigue, chronic infections, sensitivity to cold, dry skin, and bone destruction.

The body can rid itself of extraneous acidity in one of two ways. It can either release acid through bodily functions such perspiration, respiration, or urination. Otherwise it can neutralize the acid by utilizing its alkaline resources. If the body does not rid itself of this extra acid, it will then be stored in the body and converted into fat.

I see so many people struggle with weight loss and all too often completely overlook this potential acid element. Your body can't break down stored acidic fat without the addition of more alkaline foods, so just eating smaller quantities of the same acidic foods may not effectively lead to weight loss. Since acidic foods also contribute to lethargy, this only cyclically contributes to the inability to shed pounds. If you want to lose weight and shift your body back to its natural state, alter the pH levels of the foods you eat. Surprisingly a lot of the things which we consume that taste acidic, in reality are not. Taste alone is really not a good determinant. For example, while lemon would be seemingly acidic, it actually has an alkaline effect once entering the body. That's one of the reasons that lemon water can be so refreshing. Briefly look over the following lists. Try to incorporate more alkaline foods into your diet whenever possible, while avoiding the over-consumption of those that are acidic. Ideally you want approximately 60% of your food intake to be alkaline.

Alkaline Forming: Alfalfa Sprouts, Almonds, Apples, Avocados, Bananas, Beets, Blackberries, Cantaloupe, Carrots, Celery, Cherries, Chili Peppers, Chives, Cinnamon, Coconut, Cucumbers, Curry, Endive, Garlic, Ginger, Grapes, Grapefruit, Lemons, Lettuce, Limes, Mangos, Melons, Mint, Molasses, Okra, Olive Oil, Onions, Oranges, Peaches, Pears, Pomegranates, Pumpkins, Radishes, Raisins, Raspberries, Seaweed, Soybeans, Spinach, Spirulina, Squash, Strawberries, Stevia, Tofu, Tomatoes, Water Chestnuts, Watermelon, and Whey Protein Powder.

Acid Forming: Almond Milk, Aspartame, Barley, Beef, Beer, Bread, Butter, Cheese, Chicken, Chocolate, Coffee, Corn, Cranberries, Eggs, Fish, Flour, Ham, Honey, Horseradish, Ice Cream, Ketchup, Lamb, Liquor, Lobster, Oatmeal, Pasta, Peanuts, Peas, Pecans, Pistachios, Pork, Rice, Rye, Sauerkraut, Shrimp, Sugar, Tapioca, Turkey, Wheat, and Wine.

So why do we discuss alkalinity in a book on raw food? It's because the raw diet tends to be very alkaline. Many consider this factor to be one of its greatest strengths. It may also potentially shed light on why rawists tend to have more energy as well as a tendency to maintain a more ideal body weight.

If you want to perform a little science experiment at home to find out your body's current pH level, try the following. Go to your local health food store and purchase some pH test strips (also known as litmus paper). pH strips allow you to test your urine sample and determine the pH level of your body. If your sample comes back with a result of less than 6.5 pH, you should certainly try to lessen your acid intake. It may mean that your body is overwhelmed and not excreting the excess acidity optimally. For testing purposes you may want to go out and get a fast food combo meal and then take the test. Record the result. Then a couple of days later detox your body with all raw foods, especially coconut water and leafy greens. Take the test again. Were the results any different?

Alkaline Water

A pH range is not limited to foods you eat, but also pertinent when it comes to the water you drink. You can buy filtration systems that are capable of converting regular tap water into its more alkaline form. Alkaline water is usually ionized with a negative charge, filtered, and then micro-clustered with the ideal pH balance that the body craves. Micro-clustering makes water seem wetter. Sounds crazy, right? Okay, let me explain. As you know water is composed of H20, two hydrogen and one oxygen atoms. These H20 water molecules then cluster together. Tap water has particularly large clusters typically ranging between ten to fifteen molecules on average. When water undergoes electrolysis these clusters are then broken down into a smaller size, usually around 1/3 of the original cluster. As a result these water molecules can penetrate the body more quickly and efficiently. Since your body is using more of the water it takes in, you will micturate less frequently.

Alkaline water has many acclaimed benefits. Most importantly, it has the ability to neutralize the body's acidity from stress and poor diet, fighting acidosis. Many diseases are related to elevated levels of acidity, such as acid reflux disease, inflammation, heart disease, high cholesterol, and obesity. Alkaline water can help flush out toxins and eliminate acidic-loaded cells that have been converted into fat, which will help you attain your ideal body weight. Plus the hydroxyl ions in alkaline water are an antioxidant and can reduce premature aging by eliminating free radicals.

Acidic water isn't completely useless; it is just not intended for human consumption. It can help the overall look and feel of your skin when mixed into bath water. (Meanwhile alkaline water should be used on your scalp as it will help strengthen, detangle, and shine your hair while locking in hydration.) Acidic water is also a natural astringent. You can gargle it to clear up bacteria. It even works as a disinfectant on minor cuts, while speeding up recovery time. It can help eliminate acne and eczema. Plus it's even known to promote the healing of sunburn. A lesser known use is its effectiveness as a household cleaning agent. Even though it has all of these amazing properties, you still don't want to drink the stuff.

Okay, so if acidic water shouldn't be consumed, are there any adverse effects to drinking alkaline water? There can be, but only if you are already over alkaline. In reality this is practically unheard of since almost all of us are over-acidic. Japan has been commonly using alkaline water for quite a while. Their results are mixed. There are diehard advocates and skeptics. There is no evidence that it hurts you, but its therapeutic claims have not exactly been substantiated beyond a doubt. The role that alkaline water plays in one's overall health is still being discovered.

Final Words

The meals of our grandparent's generation were relatively alkaline. Take-out food was not the norm and sodas were a treat. Today just about everything we consume is acidic. As drastically as our diets have changed, we hardly ever discuss the effects of alkalinity. Anyone struggling with weight loss needs to take pH into account when dieting.

If you want to take alkalinity even more seriously then you can purchase a mechanism that will microcluster your tap water and ensure that it reaches the optimal pH balance. Some people out there dismiss alkaline water as being silly, since the human body will convert water to meet its needs. After all, you don't see people keeling over because they couldn't handle the tap water. These skeptics believe that the companies selling alkaline water and/or filtration machines are generating propaganda. Others swear by the stuff, considering it to be nothing short of a miracle. Many believe that the drug industry doesn't want you to find out how wonderful you can feel with such an easy and quick fix.

Personally, I lie somewhere in the middle. I am a believer but not a fanatic. I started out as a major skeptic, until I decided to give the stuff a chance. A friend of mine had given me a few gallons of pH balanced water to try for a week. I thought it was silly, but figured I had nothing to lose. Upon taking the first sip I noticed the water tasted better, it had an almost silky texture. In fact, the micro-clusters were smooth and quite discernible, much to my surprise. Regardless,

I didn't put much faith into it as having any healing qualities. But since the water tasted delicious, I immediately began drinking more.

The taste and texture is far superior to regular old water, so for that reason alone it is worth buying. If it leads you to drink more water, it has done its job at improving your health. Is it miracle water? I honestly don't know. But I can say that my skin and hair have never felt better. It's obvious that I am a converted believer, but I do not necessarily advocate that everyone run out and buy a filtration system. You need to try it first, and see if it's something that seems beneficial to you. You can purchase a couple of gallons from your local health food store and see what you think. Alkaline bottled water is starting to become more mainstream and is now being stocked in many gas stations and quick marts.

4 THE ART OF JUICING

Juicing is incredible. If you have not yet discovered it, go now. Run to your local kitchen appliance retailer and buy a juicer immediately. Fresh made juices are scrumptious, simple, and one of the best things you can do for your body. It amazes me that so few people today have a juice machine. It should be a staple in every kitchen. Juicing is great for everyone, from children to senior citizens. It is an effective method of easily consuming all of the nutrients you need, while enabling your body to help cure itself of certain ailments naturally.

Juicing is a sub-category of the raw diet. As much or as little of your raw diet can be in the form of juice depending on your preference and taste. It is the easiest way to consume plentiful servings of fruits and vegetables, plus all of their micronutrients. Practically every nutritionist out there is going to advocate you eating a serving of six to eight fruits and veggies per day. This would be darn near impossible for most of us, if it weren't for juicing. In fact with just two juices a day you can easily make over 50% of your diet raw.

So, what is juicing? Macerating, also known as squeezing, the liquid content out of fruits and vegetables. You can do so either by hand (although difficult and questionably even feasible) or easily with an electronic juicer. Sure you can buy juice from a store, but there are a few problems with that...

1) You will probably be consuming globs of high fructose corn syrup. Read your labels!!! Watch out for anything called "nectar", it's likely a highly-sugared and diluted form of fruit juice. You might as well be guzzling down a soda.

2) They are inundated with nasty chemicals (for coloring and preservation).

3) You may be able to purchase enough fruit juices, but likely struggle with finding a variety of vegetable juices out there. With your own juices, the possibilities and combinations are endless.

4) Store bought juices are typically diluted to cut down on costs.

5) You won't be getting the skin and pulp which is where so much of the nutritional content is contained. Plus you are also losing out on the fiber.

6) Fresh juices contain all of their living enzymes. Store bought juices have typically undergone pasteurization. In the process their enzymes are destroyed.

Juicing is really a do-it-yourself art. There are people out there, juicarians, who have replaced food altogether with juice. I do not advocate this lifestyle choice. Mainly because I do not believe our bodies were made solely to drink liquids. We need solid foods to keep our bodies strong. However I do believe that we should integrate juices into our normal diets (whatever those may be). Ideally I suggest adding two juices to your routine daily. I like to enjoy a juice in the morning for breakfast and then one in the afternoon as a snack. It's a great pick me up a little after lunch when you're starting to feel sluggish. Juice can easily replace your coffee habit (if you want it to, that is).

Why should you start juicing?

I would immediately counter this by saying, why not? It's delicious! But let's look at some of the actual reasons why juicing is so advantageous...

Allow nutrients to easily penetrate your system. You can actually absorb all of those nutrients that your body has been eliminating as waste. Years of poor dietary choices have left our bodies worn and less easily capable of proper digestion.

Enjoy your daily recommended five servings of fruits and vegetables effortlessly. Downing a glass of juice is fairly simple and you can easily consume several serving sizes.

Appease finicky eaters. Many people love certain fruits and vegetables juiced, that they would have otherwise abhorred. This was the case for me with beets. I despised them in their natural state. Sure, I knew that they were good for me, but simply were not worth the torture. Strangely when mixed into a juice, I found beets to be delicious!!! You never know what your new found delight might be. (PS- This is a great way to get kids to finally eat their vegetables.)

Keep your carbohydrate and calorie intake low. Yet you get to enjoy a high concentration of vitamins and minerals.

Improve your pH balance. Dark green vegetables, in particular, are extremely alkaline.

Stay regular. Fruit is a phenomenal source of fiber.

Suppress your appetite. Hold your body over with some nutrients instead of empty calories.

Get hydrated. Few of us drink the recommended six to eight cups of water per day. Instead we down sugary beverages that dehydrate us further. Fruits contain an extremely high pure water content.

Inundate your body with antioxidants. The chlorophyll found in some veggies is an especially powerful detoxifying agent.

Obtain enzymes. Fresh juices are packed with them. These enzymes are like fuel for your body. Ease digestion while reducing premature aging.

Heal more quickly. When your cells are operating optimally, your body heals the way nature intended.

Lower your bad cholesterol. A diet rich in fruits and vegetables will help you lower your LDL levels (bad cholesterol) while raising your HDL levels (good cholesterol).

The Practical Challenges

You do need to buy a quality juicer. So it does take an initial financial investment. Then once you buy your juicer you have to cut and juice your items and then clean the machine afterwards. Do not leave your juicer dirty! Mold growth is nasty and does happen. Think of a piece of old nasty fruit lying around. You will quickly defeat your healthy eating habit if you fail to keep things sanitary. Juicing is really not that much effort when you compare it to cooking a meal, but it does take some time nonetheless.

You should only juice when you're ready to drink. Don't make your juices in advance for the sake of convenience. Most of the contents are highly perishable. Think about what happens when you slice an apple and leave it on the counter. After a while, it begins to turn brown. Would you want to drink that brown juice? Probably not. You should juice your drinks right before consuming them. This can be a challenge since you may not always be around your juicer at a convenient time.

A Rainbow of Benefits

Typically speaking the following colors of produce are indicative of the following health benefits. These characteristics not true of every single fruit and/or vegetable and are somewhat of a generalization, but interesting nonetheless. The more color you incorporate into your diet, the better. Except, maybe for Skittles, those don't count. The more vibrant the color of the fruit or vegetable, the greater the antioxidant content. Deep, rich pigments signify a strong nutritional value.

Yellow/Gold - Yellow is often a sign of beta carotene, which helps your body produce vitamin A. These foods are beneficial for your skin and eye health. According to a study by the University of St. Andrews, the yellowish-red pigmentation from produce can even be absorbed by fat cells, giving your complexion a youthful grow.

Blue/Purple – Many blue foods contain anthocyanins. They are rich in antioxidants and can help eliminate cancer-causing free radicals.

Red - Red foods may possess lycopene, which can reduce your risk of cancer and pre-mature aging. The reds are also beneficial to your bloodstream, preventing clots and improving circulation.

Green - Green means a boost to your immunity. It usually signifies chlorophyll, which aids detoxification and tissue generation.

White - White foods can help lower cholesterol. They also may aid in preventing certain types of cancers and regulating blood pressure.

Fruit Juice - A Natural Sugar Rush

Fruits do contain a certain amount of fructose and glucose, also known as sugars. Often people going raw are concerned that the sugars found in fruits, and even vegetables, will be harmful to their health. It is good to remain cautious of not raising your blood sugar levels too high when eating raw, but I think we often forget just how much sugar is in processed foods. It seems like every label I read these days has a walloping sugar content. When we compare this artificial sugar to the sweetness found in natural foods, it seems miniscule. In order to best understand the effect that natural sugar has on our bodies first we need to become familiar with some basic terminology.

Fructose and Glucose are simple sugars, both monosaccharides that are relatively simple for your body to process. Fruits may contain a small amount of both and your body can convert these simple sugars into energy. While the two probably are fundamentally more similar than different, there are some ways to differentiate the two forms of the compound known as $C_6H_{12}O_6$. The two slightly differ in their molecular structure. Glucose, unlike fructose, requires insulin to break it down. Fructose is slowly released into the body, and doesn't cause that sudden sugar rush. Glucose is sometimes called "dextrose" by marketing experts who believe that glucose holds a negative connotation amongst consumers. Glucose really isn't such a bad thing though. If you are active, your body actually needs it for energy, but in moderation. It's vital to your system, but you need to manage its release (aka: your blood sugar levels).

High Fructose Corn Syrup is made up of 55% fructose and 45% glucose. While fructose and glucose in moderation, and in their natural state, are not all that harmful, high fructose corn syrup is a completely different thing. It is an artificially derived sweetener that is heavily utilized due to its cheap cost. Its placed in just about everything these days, some examples include barbecue sauce, cereal, bread, yogurt, deli meat, ice cream, crackers, ketchup, salad dressing, and most notoriously... soda. The America consumption of high fructose corn syrup is skyrocketing at unprecedented levels, and negative publicity is finally arousing some consumer concern.

The corn syrup industry is constantly trying to tell us that sugar is sugar. They claim that it is no different from any other type of sugar out there. However a lot of speculation traces high fructose corn syrup to be linked to obesity. In 2010 the Corn Refiners Association petitioned the FDA to call high fructose corn syrup, simply "corn syrup" to avoid its negative connotation amongst consumers.

Even worse than high fructose corn syrup, is **aspartame**, the stuff in diet soda. Personally I'd probably rather drink rat poison. Oh wait, it is rat poison. Okay, not really. But it is very, very bad for you. Various studies amongst humans and lab rats show that it causes brain damage, disturbances in neuroendoctrine function, memory loss, brain tumors, mood disorders, headaches, insomnia, seizures, blindness, accelerated aging, nausea, weight gain, premature birth in pregnant women, hypoglycemia, thyroid problems, and asthma. And that's just the beginning.

The ingestion of aspartame leads to the formation of methanol. Methanol causes headaches, vertigo, numbness, inner-ear disturbances, nausea, vision trouble, heart problems, pancreatic inflammation, neuritis, chills, and conjunctivitis, amongst many other horrible problems. Even more terrifying is that methanol converts into formaldehyde. Yes, the stuff used for embalming dead people. Chronic exposure to formaldehyde leads to even more trouble. It causes immune system dysfunction, irreversible gene damage, and changes to your nervous system. Still don't want to give up your Diet Coke? There's more. I'm only listing some of the ninety problems associated with aspartame. The phenylalanine in aspartame causes a decrease in serotonin levels, schizophrenia, seizures, uterine polyps, and brain cancer. The airline industry is filled with articles discouraging pilots from consuming it. Comforting, eh?

You may be wondering just how this stuff is allowed by the FDA. Simple, there are studies out there that say the contrary, that it poses no risk to human beings. Aspartame has been the world's most commonly used alternative sweetener ever since its introduction in 1981. Not that long ago, really. It is a common held belief by many consumer groups and doctors that the initial approval of this substance was fraudulent, but the government and manufacturers of the product refuse to examine the matter further.

When people develop adverse reactions to this stuff it's from consuming it over a long period of time. You don't down one packet of artificial sweetener and develop cancer. It's a long, slow drawn out process. Your physician isn't necessarily going to associate that your current ailment has been caused by aspartame, even if it has. It may very well be the root of the problem, but medically speaking we treat symptoms. It may take a few generations to understand the long term effects that this stuff has on the human population. The best advice I can give you, even if you take nothing else away from this book, is to avoid aspartame like the plague. It has no nutritional value whatsoever and can potentially do your body so much harm. This billion dollar industry thrives, and even has unknowing masses of the population fooled into thinking they are actually providing their body with a healthy alternative to sugar.

If you want sugar, just consume good old sugar. Even better yet, go with stevia. And as the best possible alternative, do what us hardcore raw foodies do… use fruits to give recipes a natural sweetness. This will help regulate your blood sugar. **The Glycemic Index** is used to rank how fast and to what degree foods will raise your blood sugar levels. Remaining conscious and careful of this can help prevent diabetes, certain cancers, heart disease, high cholesterol, and obesity.

Your body has a limited capacity to store sugar. Once you exceed your body's allotted intake the fructose present begin to turn into **triglycerides**. These triglycerides are then released into your blood stream where they can lead to all sorts of adverse health effects, such as weight gain. To best moderate your triglyceride levels eat fruits that are high in fiber and that do not contain high levels of fructose.

When we consume fructose, it heads to our liver for processing. If we have too much fructose in our system, our body starts converting it into a fat and increases our triglyceride count. When we consume glucose on the other hand, **insulin** is released into the bloodstream to help regulate it. A little insulin secretion is necessary to help the glucose process into the body and provide energy. Too much insulin however, especially over a prolonged period, is harmful.

Grapefruit is an excellent choice of fruit for diabetics since it can help stabilize insulin levels. If you are diabetic or suffer from blood sugar related issues you need to be rather cautious of the type of fruit and amounts you incorporate into your diet. You should avoid an overconsumption of grapes, watermelon, pineapple, and oranges, to name a few. You can still enjoy fruits in general, but find those which are high in fiber and low in glucose. Fiber helps slow the rate at which sugar enters the bloodstream. You can easily see which fruits and veggies are lowest in sugar content by consulting a glycemic index.

In general, an overindulgence in natural sugars from eating fresh fruits and vegetables is not something the average person needs to be much concerned about. Although everyone, whether cautious about their sugar levels or not, should avoid canned fruits, store bought juices, and dried fruits whenever possible. They contain an unnecessarily high sugar content. Canned fruits are usually soaked in some sort of sugary syrup and preservatives. Store bought juices are watered down and often high in added sugar. And finally, dried fruit has a high sugar content for its size. It's easy to unknowingly overindulge. If you were eating the same serving size you would with real fruit, the sugar content is no longer an issue. Do be careful though, because some of the companies that sell dried fruit, do add sugar.

Final Words

There is no easier way to go raw than by incorporating fruit and vegetable juices into your diet. Aim to drink at least two juices per day. Normal sized portions of fruits and vegetables should not adversely affect your blood sugar if you are a healthy adult. Those concerned with their blood sugar levels can still enjoy juicing, but will have to ensure that they are selecting fruits and vegetables that are high in fiber while low in glucose.

5 FRUIT GUIDE

We all know that fruit is good for us, even essential, yet oddly enough as a society we simply just don't eat enough of it. While modern science has confirmed just how beneficial fruit is for our bodies, our grandparents never needed this validation. They intuitively trusted the healing properties of the proper diet. Sure you can pop a vitamin but there are two flaws in that plan. First, you could never replicate all of the various types of nutrients. The phytonutrients of a supplement could never compare to that of a natural food. And secondly, your body does not absorb or assimilate the benefits of a pill in the same way. You're only getting a fraction of the benefits. Despite what we'd like to believe, vitamins are not a quick fix for poor dietary choices. Your best bet is to eat a varied diet of natural foods.

The right foods can help prevent disease and even promote healing when ill. Most of the fruits on this list will help prevent cancer, fight heart disease, and lower your cholesterol. Be that as it may, before attempting to cure yourself of any disease(s) consult with your physician. I do not advocate using foods alone to replace medicine, but to be used as a preventative measure and in conjunction with your doctor's proscribed regiment in healing. Keep in mind that new studies and discoveries are being made every day. I used to joke about the flux of chocolate and wine, they seem to be good for you one day and bad the next. Luckily I have yet to hear of any studies showing any fruit or vegetable to be adverse to your health. However we must realize that the world of nutrition is in constant motion. I have made every attempt to provide the most current and accurate information possible. This list is by no means all-inclusive, in foods or benefits, but it should give you a fun foundation for reference.

Acai: Acai berries are highly perishable. As a result, it is challenging to find these berries perfectly ripe when outside of their growing area. Despite their rarity, acai seem to be the buzzword of health food fans everywhere. They are a superfood and their fame absolutely justified. Acai are said to do all of the following… slow aging, aid brain development, jumpstart weight loss, improve circulation, combat cancer, promote heart health, improve sleep, increase concentration, and assist with digestion. All of these things occur because acai berries are loaded with omega-3 fatty acids, vitamins A/B/C/E, minerals, phytonutrients, fiber, and antioxidants. That's a whole lot of goodness in a little package.

Apple: There may just be some credence to that "apple a day" adage. Although perhaps we neglected to add that it keeps the dentist away as well. The acidic content of apple juice serves as an antiseptic and can help prevent tooth decay. But that's not all. They are a head to toe boost for the human body. Apples are beneficial to our nervous systems, aid in digestion, relieve asthma, lower bad cholesterol, and help maintain heart health. The phloridzin and boron found in apples can strengthen bones, while their quercertin content may fight against the free radical damage that can lead to Alzheimer's. Plus, this very same quercertin combined with another flavonoid called naringin has shown to significantly reduce one's risk of lung cancer. Recent studies give us reason to believe that apples reduce one's risk of breast and liver cancers as well. Another study in Brazil found that women who ate either an apple or a pear on a daily basis lost more weight than those who did not. If you enjoy juicing its super simple to integrate apples into your diet, as they make an instant and natural sweetener to most vegetable juices. You can add apple to just about everything. Enjoying an apple for breakfast can actually provide you with more energy than drinking a cup of coffee. With over 7,000 different varieties out there, what's your excuse not to have one? No longer the forbidden fruit, enjoy this healthy pleasure.

Apricot: It's not at all surprising that apricots are high in beta-carotene, due to their coloring, but what you might not know is that they are also plentiful sources of vitamin C, potassium, and magnesium. Apricots are very good for your eyes and lungs. When juiced they don't produce a lot of liquid, but the nectar that you squeeze out of each one, will be well worth it. It's quite fitting that apricot means "precious" in Latin.

Avocado: Avocados are a staple for raw foodies due to their protein content. They make a satisfying and hearty meal in a diet that has a tendency to veer on the light side. You can eat an avocado on its own garnished with a splash of lime juice, salt, and pepper or integrate it into recipes. While scrumptious in its solid form, you should not juice an avocado. Their pulp will jam up your juicer. This stubborn pulp however, is where all of the nutrients lie.

An avocado contains palmitoleic, oleic, and linoleic acids. These acids are great because they are one of the key benefits to the acclaimed Mediterranean diet. They will lower your LDL (bad cholesterol) levels and increase your HDL (good cholesterol) levels. Avocados are also high in fiber, tannins, potassium (often twice as much as a banana), iron, copper, manganese, magnesium, and vitamins A/C/K. In summation, avocados will help remove oxygen-depriving free radicals from your body, reducing your risk of many cancers and pre-mature aging. Plus, they are incredibly alkalizing. Avocados mostly contain a monounsaturated fat that can be burned for energy. There is a downside to all of this though. Avocados contain something called persin which is dangerous for pets. There are plenty of meals to be shared with Fido, especially when eating raw and natural, but avocado dishes should be avoided.

Did You Know: *You can speed up an avocado's ripening process by placing it in a paper bag with an apple.*

Banana: I hate to break it to you, but technically speaking a banana is not really a fruit. It's actually an herb. The bundle of bananas that you buy at the store are called a hand, and then each individual banana is referred to as a finger. Their peel has a relieving effect on mosquito bites, but that's not really why people buy them. Bananas are most notorious as being a rich source of potassium. They possess many other lesser known benefits as well. They remedy heartburn by acting as a neutralizer. Bananas also contain the amino acid, tryptophan, which boosts your mood and promotes relaxation. Their high iron content combats anemia. And since they are a good source of fiber, they relieve constipation. Bananas are another one of those things that you just should not juice. They are simply too mushy, so they'll clog your juicer. Besides, can you imagine the stringy texture? Yuck. But who cares because bananas in their raw form are a delicious treat that will enhance your mental clarity and focus.

Bell Pepper: You may be somewhat surprised to see bell peppers listed under fruit. Their savory flavor can be deceiving. When we think of fruits, we tend to think sweet. Bell peppers prove that this is not always the case. They contain traces of capsaicin which an anti-inflammatory, anti-carcinogenic, anti-diabetic, and anti-bacterial. While normally a great food choice, avoid bell peppers if you suffer from a gastro-esophageal reflux condition.

Red and yellow peppers are preferable to green peppers when it comes to nutritional value. The red and yellow varieties have incredibly higher concentration of vitamins A/C. While the green varieties aren't as potent they still contain about twice the vitamin C content of an orange. According to a study performed by Cornell University, red pepper juice may inhibit the growth of nitrosamines, known carcinogens. Red peppers also contain lycopene which can prevent cervical and prostate cancers. Yellow varieties promote healthy skin, strong teeth, and wound healing. All bell peppers, regardless of their color, have a good deal of fiber, beta carotene, folic acid, and vitamins B6. They help keep your blood vessels in optimal shape and protect against heart disease. Bell peppers boost your immunity while reducing some of the risks incurred by smoking, such as emphysema.

Did You Know: *Bell peppers can even come in purple.*

Blackberry: There is something pretty funky about blackberry juice. No, it's not the taste. But that it can help prevent brain aging. This isn't something we are riddled with anxiety about, since we're usually more preoccupied with concealing crow's feet. Brain age is an overlooked, yet important factor. The high ellagic acid content of blackberries also make them an excellent cancer preventer. On the downside, blackberries can be sort of pricey and spoil quickly.

Blueberry: Blueberries are another superfood. They are loaded with phytoflavinoids, vitamin C, potassium, and antioxidants. Remember the darker the berry, the higher the antioxidant content. Blueberries lower your risk of heart disease and cancer. They also have an anti-inflammatory property thereby counteracting a host of inflammation related ailments.

Black Current: These berries are not all that common in the U.S. as they are native to Europe and Asia. Even though the name suggests they would be black, they come in several color varieties. Opt for the black ones though; they have the greatest concentration of nutrients. Black currents contain iron, vitamin a/b1/b5/b6/c, anthocyanins (an antioxidant found in dark colored fuits), copper, phosphorous, calcium, potassium, magnesium, and manganese. They are good for your blood and bones, while preventing inflammation and eliminating free radicals.

Cantaloupe: Members of the cantaloupe family include pumpkin, squash, and cucumber (just to drop a few A-list names). Cantaloupe is enriched with one of the greatest amounts of vitamin A of all fruits. Vitamin A is beneficial to your health as it is an antioxidant which is good for your eyesight. It keeps your mucous membranes in order while preventing lung and oral cancers. Plus it's fantastic for radiant looking skin. What is not to love? Oh and cantaloupes happen to contain beta carotene, zeaxanthin, and potassium.

Cherry: Just as with blueberries, the darker the cherry, the higher the antioxidant content. Darker cherries contain higher traces of anthocyanins, which block two types of enzymes and are thereby deemed an anti-inflammatory. Cherries are known to treat muscle pain, gout, arthritis, and a number of inflammation related problems. A study by the University of Michigan confirmed that inflammation, as well as cholesterol and triglyceride levels, were all reduced in lab rats with cherry consumption. It's no real surprise as the medicinal properties of cherries go way back. The ancient Greeks used them to heal scabs. Today we also know that they do wonders for the heart, kidneys, and skin. According to a recent USA Today article, the FDA is somewhat at odds with the cherry industry. This is not because eating cherries has any adverse effects, rather it's because the FDA does not want the industry touting the health benefits of cherries without them being first approved as a drug. Is this an attempt by Big Pharma to control the market or a matter of public safety? You decide.

Coconut: Coconuts can help kill bacteria, protozoa, viruses, lice, fungi, and tapeworms. They can relieve, heal, or prevent symptoms from gallbladder disease, kidney stones, eczema, fatigue, nausea, inflammation, nail fungus, cancer, dementia, osteoporosis, anxiety, cystic fibrosis, hemorrhoids, allergies, asthma, epilepsy, dandruff, hot flashes, ulcers, and diabetes. That's quite a list and far from complete. Best of all, coconut consumption has no harmful side effects, unlike conventional medicine. I'm not saying that you should forego your medicine for any of the aforementioned ailments; rather I want to point out that coconut seems to be a beneficial addition to your diet. If you want to speed up your metabolism and help your body absorb more precious nutrients, coconut is the way to go. Their oil has long been notorious for its medicinal properties amongst the Pacific Island population, and current research is starting to confirm many of these claims.

Coconut water is really catching on as a popular mainstream beverage as of late. Replace your soda intake with coconut water; all of the flavored blends make it an easy swap. Plus, it's a much healthier alternative. Coconuts are nature's Gatorade. They make for an electrolyte loaded beverage. Plus, coconut water helps alkalize your body.

Did You Know: *Mixing together some coconut oil and peppermint extract makes a potent insect repellent. It even hydrates your skin at the same time. If you forget to apply some repellent and get bit, no worries, apply some coconut oil to the affected area after the fact for some instant itch relief.*

Cranberry: Native Americans often used cranberries as medicine. Their juice is a notoriously used cure to help clear up a urinary tract infection, but cranberries are capable of a great deal more. In fact, they are even powerful enough to help prevent an E-coli infection by inhibiting the attachment of bacteria. They increase good and lower bad cholesterol levels. Plus, cranberries are said to prevent gum disease and ulcers. As with any food, moderation is important. Over inundating your body with cranberries can thin your blood when taken with certain medications. This is rare, but should be cautioned nonetheless.

Did You Know: *Cranberries have also been called 'bounceberries' since they bounce when ripe.*

Cucumber: Modern society often misconstrues cucumbers as a vegetable, but they actually belong to the fruit family on a technicality. Their seeds are contained within their centers. Cucumber juice is a fantastic choice for newbies. It's mild in flavor, but surprisingly delicious. It aids in weight loss and helps regulate blood sugar levels of those suffering from diabetes. Cucumber juice can be a mild diuretic while a strong source of electrolytes. Plus, the vitamin K content of cucumbers may help fight Alzheimer's, by limiting potential neuron damage.

Durian Fruit: In my experience, the people who have tried durian druit either have a passionate love or deeply seeded hatred for this peculiar fruit. It's distinct. Not only in taste, but also, in its makeup. It contains tryptophan which is used to treat a huge list of things such as insomnia, anxiety, depression, suppress appetite, nightmares, bulimia, Parkinson's Disease, Obsessive Compulsive Disorder, and migraines.

Eggplant: Another surprise on the fruit list. Studies in Brazil have found eggplant to positively treat high cholesterol. The anthocyanins in eggplant may also protect against cancer, neurological damage, and aging.

Did You Know: *Eggplant actually contains small traces of nicotine. Do not be all too concerned though. The concentration is so minuscule that it should not discourage you from enjoying these surprise fruits, which are quite nutritious.*

Gac: Repulsive name, scrumptious fruit. Gac contains one of the highest lycopene and beta carotene concentrations on earth. It's used to treat eye, skin, reproductive, prostate, and heart health.

Goji Berry: These bright colored berries help prevent aging, certain cancers, high cholesterol, and heart disease. While goji berry supplements are being peddled by holistic healing advocates, how these supplements compare to their real counterpart, in terms of effectiveness, is still being researched.

Gooseberry: These guys are closely related to their cousin, black currents. They, too, have high traces of anthocyanins and flavones which fight pre-mature aging, several cancers, inflammation, and keep your neurological system in working order.

Grapefruit: As with many of the other fruits, grapefruits keep you regular, decrease your risk of cancer, and can help alkalinize your body. But one of the wonderfully unique properties of grapefruit is that it is a fantastic choice for those who have diabetes since it contains an antioxidant called naringenin. Also, their salicylic acid content may prevent arthritis. And the pectin of grapefruit may help lower elevated cholesterol levels.

Grape: When grapes are consumed regularly they have an interesting cooling effect on the body. Darker grapes contain anthocyanins while the lighter colored varieties contain a greater amount of tannins. You can't go wrong. All grapes are rich in resveratrol which reduces your risk of stroke. According to Dr. Rajesh Agarwal, of the University of Colorado Cancer Center, when grape seed extract was given to mice it reduced the growth of certain cancers upto 67%. Professional journal, *Carcinogenesis*, has explained that there is evidence to suggest that grape seed oil can destroy cancer cells that target the head and neck area. For a more everyday application you can juice just a handful of grapes to help relieve constipation. Just don't put them in the microwave, they explode. (Don't ask me how I know this.)

Did You Know: *Raisins are a better source of iron than grapes.*

Green Bean: I would have lost this bet. Green beans are a fruit, not a vegetable. They are a mislabeled nutritional powerhouse. Green beans are high in folates and therefore beneficial during pregnancy. They contain zeaxanthin which promotes eye health. Their dietary fiber is great for lowering bad cholesterol and maintaining colon health. Plus, green beans contain a natural insulin that is good for diabetics.

Guava: Guavas are a superfruit that can help the body heal all sorts of ailments. These fruits can relieve constipation, help with collagen production, prevent certain cancers, help cure dysentery, improve skin tone, lower high blood pressure, remedy scurvy, provide relief from the common cold, keep heart-rate regular, maintain the integrity of the bloodstream, increase semen production, and rid your body of intestinal worms. Their high concentrations of vitamins A/C and lycopene are soaked up like a sponge by the human body.

Honeydew: Of all the melons, honeydew surprisingly has the highest sugar content. Don't worry about it though; this North American melon staple makes up for this minor downside in nutritional value. Honeydew are rich in potassium, vitamin C, and fiber. Regular consumption of this melon can lower your risk of age-related macular degeneration, certain cancers, stroke, heart disease, and diabetes. Honeydew juice is a superb anti-aging tool that aids skin regeneration.

Kiwi: Since kiwis are high in vitamins A, C, and E they can help you prevent and/or get over the common cold and flu. Their flavonoids and carotenoids help reduce the risk of cancer. Recent studies are showing that kiwis may even prevent blood clots. Kiwi juice can be somewhat tart so be sure to pair it with something relatively sweet

Kumquat: Unlike its relatives, the orange and the tangerine, the kumquat can be eaten in its entirety (peel included). Low in calories, high in nutrients, and drenched in sweetness these fruits are a delicacy. They are loaded with flavonoid antioxidants and essential oils. Kumquats can help eliminate free-radicals.

Lemon: You may see people squeeze a dash of lemon into their water and think they are crazy. Some find it to be an acquired taste, but there is something remarkably addictive to it once you get in the habit. Fresh squeezed lemon juice helps you maintain the proper alkalinity. I discourage the use of store bought lemon juice. It's pasteurized and experiences a similar effect to cooked vegetables; it's missing much of the good stuff. Fresh squeezed lemon juice helps you hydrate, detoxify, and boost your immunity. It's used to aid weight loss, inflammation, cramps, and several skin conditions. Interestingly enough it is also a known sedative and can even help prevent vomiting. If you have a gassy tummy, try a little lemon water. It's a quick and successful fix. The acid content of lemons can help kill bacteria. They make an excellent cleaning agent or makeshift hand sanitizer with a hot towel.

Did You Know: *The tradition of serving a lemon wedge with a piece of fish originated in the Middle Ages, when it was believed that a dash of lemon would dissolve any potentially swallowed fish bones.*

Lime: The lime is very similar to its sibling, the lemon, in nutritional composition. However, they differ in color and taste. It's a preference thing. It does have one thing over the lemon, though, something called limonene. Limonene is a phytochemical that helps relieve heartburn.

Loquat: These fruits can be described as similar to an apple. One thing worth noting about loquats is that they contain pectin. Pectin binds to toxicities in the colon, and can help reduce your odds of contracting colon cancer. Pectin also helps reduce LDL cholesterol levels. In history, loquats have been considered a sedative and used to calm a nervous stomach. People have even utilized this fruit in certain cases to counteract depression naturally.

Caution: *Loquat seeds can be toxic, because of their amygdalin. Clearly, I do not recommend eating the seeds. Interestingly enough, many urban legends say these seeds are a remarkably powerful cancer cure. Considering where the studies lie at the present time, I suggest you wait. Do not take any chances with these seeds until we have more information.*

Lychee: Lychee fruit help your nails and hair grow and your skin regenerate. They are a beautician's delight. Lychee contain antioxidants, beta carotene, phosphorous, calcium, magnesium, vitamins B/C, and potassium. They are a natural diuretic that increase your body's overall wellbeing.

Mango: Research is starting to show that mangoes can protect against leukemia, colon, breast, and prostate cancers because of their polyphenolic antioxidant compounds. They also improve skin health, digestion, sex drive, and memory. Moreover, they are rich sources of potassium, vitamins A/B6/C/E, and copper.

Mangosteen: Being low in calories and high in dietary fiber, these fruits very popular amongst dieters. They are great for heart health and the immune system. Practitioners of holistic medicine use mangosteens to cure infection and reduce inflammation. Modern research confirms these practitioner's beliefs and gives us reason to think that mangosteens are beneficial in preventing diabetes, vertigo, anxiety, cataracts, glaucoma, gum disease, kidney stones, and Alzheimer's disease. Plus, their polysaccharides can inhibit cancer and bacteria growth. I imagine we'll be hearing a lot more about mangosteens in the near future.

Mulberry: These somewhat less notorious fruits may potentially combat cancer, aging, diabetes, and inflammation. They contain zeaxanthin (good for the retina of your eyes) as well as resveratrol (good for your blood), along with vitamins A/C/E.

Olive: While typically utilized in a fashion similar to a vegetable, they are actually a fruit. Attention is almost always focused on their oil, and rightfully so, but we shouldn't neglect the olive itself. The oleuropein and hydroxytyrosol phytonutrients contained within olives effectively combat osteoporosis and cancer. They are an anti-inflammatory and loaded with antioxidants. Sure olives contain a high fat content, but this is a good fat. One our body needs and craves. This fat has the ability to lower bad cholesterol and reduce the risk of heart disease. Olives can also relieve a cough, fight infections, and stop diarrhea.

Orange: Obviously oranges have a high Vitamin C content. We learn that from the time we are young children. But oranges have a ton of other lesser known nutritional benefits as well, such as flavonoids. They are rich in antioxidants and their white membrane contains a good deal of calcium. Orange juice is known to help boost immunity, fight cancer and heart disease, lower bad cholesterol, and combat high blood pressure.

Papaya: Papaya juice is great for the heart, liver, and spleen. It can even increase male virility. Plus the beta carotene, vitamin C/E, and enzymes within a papaya can treat inflammation and prevent cancer. Meanwhile, their antioxidant and fiber content may lower cholesterol, prevent heart disease, and reduce your risk of stroke. Tea made from papaya leaves is consumed to help prevent malaria. But if you have a latex allergy beware. Papaya actually contains latex. Generally speaking, the less ripe the fruit, the greater the latex content.

Did You Know: *You can add some shine to your hair by making a papaya-yogurt mask. Leave it in for about twenty minutes and then rinse.*

Passion Fruit: Delicious and loaded with vitamins A/C, copper, magnesium, iron, phosphorous, and potassium. These fruits are an anti-inflammatory, preventer of certain cancers, and can help regulate blood pressure.

Peach: Studies show that peaches can help inhibit tumor growth and act as an antimicrobial. They are high in vitamin C, lycopene, and lutein. Even if a peach is not ripe enough to eat, it may still be perfect for juicing.

Pear: The ancient Greeks used pears as a remedy to nausea. Homer referred to them as a "gift from the gods". Even today pears are used to help treat things such as gout, gallbladder disorders, arthritis, and colitis. They are good sources of dietary fiber, vitamins, flavonoids, and minerals.

Did You Know: *Back before tobacco was popular people would smoke pear leaves.*

Persimmon: This fruit contains catechins, gallocatechins, and betullinic acid. Such compounds can prevent tumors, hemorrhages, and inflammation. The antioxidant content of a persimmon can also help slow aging.

Pineapple: When you pick up a pineapple from your local grocery store, what you probably don't realize is that it took around eighteen months for that single pineapple to grow. It's okay though, all good things are worth the wait. Pineapple is excellent for your bones and circulation. Another added bonus is that pineapple contains something called Bromelain enzymes. While the benefits of Bromelian enzymes are still being studied, they are thought to slow the growth of cancer cells, relieve sinusitis, and aid post surgery healing. Pineapple can help rid your body of trapped gas and destroy intestinal worms. Basically if there is something in your digestive system that shouldn't be there, drink a little pineapple juice to naturally help it work its way out.

Plum: Plums are a good source of fiber, potassium, iron, calcium, and magnesium. Dried plums (prunes) are commonly known for their ability to keep you regular. Their acid compounds have an anti-cancer effect. Plums, and prunes, will help keep wrinkles at bay, regulate blood sugar, and ensure your heart is pumping as it should.

Pomegranate: Pomegranates are enriched with tannins (yes, the stuff in wine), polyphenols, and anthocyanins. They have been suggested to help alleviate everything from male erectile dysfunction to the effects of aging. This superfood has a great deal of benefits. Their juice has an even higher antioxidant content than green tea. According to a study by the University of California pomegranate juice is incredibly powerful at eliminating free-radicals. This is important because free radicals can damage DNA and be related to premature aging and cancer. In another study of men undergoing prostate cancer treatments, those consuming pomegranate juice on a consistent basis required less treatment. If for no other reason, drink a nice glass of pomegranate juice to help eliminate dental plaque.

Did You Know: *The pomegranate is considered to be sacred in several of the world's major religions. In the book of Exodus it is instructed that a pomegranate be woven into the robes of Hebrew Priests. Some believe it was actually even a pomegranate, not an apple, that tempted Adam and Eve in the Garden of Eden. In the Jewish faith the pomegranate is seen as righteous since it is thought to have 613 seeds, just as the Torah has 613 commandments. The actual seed content does vary though. In the Qur'an it is said that pomegranates will be found in the garden of paradise. Then in the Hindu tradition pomegranates symbolize fertility and abundance. Holy fruit (pun intended)!!*

Pumpkin: Not only are pumpkins a fruit, but also the world's largest fruit. Pumpkins are low in calories while dense in nutrients. They are a good source of omega-3 fatty acids, beta-carotene, and vitamin E. Pumpkins control healthy mucous production, support eye and bone health, all while providing a boost to your immunity.

Raspberry: Raspberries are a phenomenal cancer fighter due to their ellagic, gallic, and salicyclic acid content. It is said that these acids can help inhibit tumor growth. Besides that, raspberries improve overall immunity, promote heart and liver health, and even help heal wounds. They have a higher antioxidant content than strawberries or blueberries. Not to brag, but they also contain anthocyanins, xylitol, quercetin, potassium, copper, manganese, magnesium, vitamins A/B/C/E/K, lutein, riboflavin, niacin, beta carotene, and zeaxanthin.

Strawberry: Strawberries seem like a cure-all to just about everything, but then again, so are most fruits and veggies. To begin, they have a good deal of fiber which regulates your cholesterol, lowers your glucose levels, and keeps you regular. Then their antioxidants fight free radicals. Next, strawberries contain folic acid. Sounds great, but what does this mean in relation to your health? Folic acid helps protect against heart disease, certain cancers, and Alzheimer's disease. Plus, it can increase male sperm count. As an added bonus, strawberries are a good source of potassium.

Did You Know: *Rubbing a strawberry on your teeth can remove surface stains. The acid found inside a strawberry can enhance the brightness of your pearly whites.*

Tangerine: Interestingly enough, a little tangerine may just have a higher vitamin C content than a big old orange. Tangerine juice is a blood-thinner and anti-inflammatory, which may help reduce the risk of heart problems and alleviate ailments such as arthritis.

Tomato: Although typically misclassified as a vegetable, a tomato is "technically-speaking" a fruit. There are actually over a thousand different types of tomato varieties out there. They are a great source of vitamins A/B/C and iron. (Opt for vine-ripened tomatoes whenever possible as they possess a greater amount of vitamin C than their counterparts.) Tomatoes can be used to aid kidney function, anemia, and constipation. Researchers out of Cornell University have identified the chlorogenic and P-courmaric acids in tomatoes to be strong cancer fighters. While seemingly acidic, tomatoes help promote alkalinity. They can also help remove unwanted sugars and be beneficial to those with diabetes. That's some good news for salsa fans. Do you enjoy your salsa blended with avocado? I hope so, because a recent study by the University of Ohio shows that when tomatoes are consumed with avocados your body can better absorb their lycopene content. Lycopene is important since it can reduce the risks of cancer and cataracts. If you're just looking to shed some unwanted pounds enjoy a nice glass of tomato juice. It is a splendid digestion aid.

Did You Know: *Tomatoes are the most consumed fruit in the United States.*

Watermelon: Oh, how I hate to break it to you, but a watermelon is another misclassified food. It's a vegetable. But this fact is still debated to this very day. Since it's so heated, we're leaving it in the fruit category. While low in fat and sodium, watermelons are a good source of vitamins A/C and potassium. They make a great mild juice to alleviate constipation and quench thirst. Don't over-do it though if you suffer from asthma, watermelons can promote unwanted coughing.

Did You Know: *Before the invention of canteens many adventurers used hollowed watermelons to carry their water.*

6 VEGETABLE GUIDE

Mother always said that you needed to finish your plate of vegetables. Probably didn't make much sense to you at the time and frankly you didn't care. Well, I have news for you. Your mom was right and so were you. As a kid it probably didn't matter all that much if you ate your plate of green peas and carrots, but a lifetime of avoiding them in going to land you in a heap of trouble. Here is a list of some common vegetables and why they are vital to your health.

Artichoke: While most often seen steamed, it is entirely possible to eat an artichoke in its raw form. Peel away the outer layers of a mature artichoke to get to the tender heart. If you opt for a younger and smaller artichoke, you will find that there will be even more parts that are edible and delectable raw. A diet consisting of artichokes is thought to help reduce cholesterol, due to the cynarin and sesquiterpene lactones. Artichokes are also believed to help gallbladder and liver conditions, while aiding in digestion and the flow of bile. Expectant mothers should particularly integrate fresh artichoke into their diets for their folic acid, magnesium, and choline content. Senior citizens should also eat their fair share of this veggie since vitamin K may help fight Alzheimer's Disease. Finally everyone can reap the benefits of the healthy acids present in artichoke which can help rid the body of harmful free-radicals. As an added bonus, artichokes have a particularly high fiber content.

Arugula: The ancients considered arugula to be an aphrodisiac. We don't put much credence on that today, but it is showing to be remarkable in aiding women's reproductive health, in cases of Human Pamplona Virus (HPV) and cervical dysplasia. The phytochemicals found in arugula also seem to be indicating positive evidence in inhibiting breast, colon, cervical, and ovarian cancers. Plus, it's super high in vitamin K and can thus support bone health.

Asparagus: One of the really cool things about asparagus is that it burns more calories to digest than you consume by eating it. It is loaded with all sorts of great vitamins and minerals. Asparagus has been used to treat irritable bowel syndrome and counter the harmful effects of radiation. It contains something called rutin which can help protect your small blood vessels and even has a cleansing effect on the blood. Plus, asparagus possesses something else called glutathione which is an anti-carcinogen. Though typically green, you can also find white and purple varieties. Diabetics and those suffering with cardio-vascular erythrism should especially integrate a healthy amount of raw asparagus into their diets.

Beet: Beets are packed with potassium, magnesium, folic acid, manganese, copper, iron, vitamin C, and phosphorous which make them powerful at providing energy and lowering blood pressure. They keep you regular and help eliminate waste that has accumulated in your body. Studies have also shown beets to be effective in improving stamina. It is worth noting that beets are high in carbohydrates.

Bok Choy: This cabbage family veggie is very low in calories, while high in minerals and nutrients. Bok Choy is wonderful for lowering cholesterol, boosting immunity, and eliminating free radicals. If these benefits don't appeal to you, well at least its fun to say.

Broccoli: It would probably be easier to talk about what broccoli doesn't do. Calorically speaking it has a similar (if not higher) calcium content to milk, so it's a fantastic option for those who are lactose intolerant. Plus, it contains double the vitamin C of an orange. Studies have shown that the selenium of broccoli has the ability to remove horrible carcinogens from the body. I'm not saying that this should replace medical treatment just yet, but imagine if simply incorporating more broccoli in to our diets would significantly reduce our risk of contracting cancer. It is said that broccoli can help eliminate abnormal cells and prevent breast cancer with its indoles. Seriously it sounds like broccoli can do us a lot of good and little harm. It's cheap, tasty, and highly nutritious.

Brussels Sprouts: Can you guess what European city these sprouts originated? The city of Brussels in Belgium of course. Sounds like something you would learn from an episode of Jeopardy. Another thing you may not be aware of is that the phytochemicals in brussels sprouts can reduce DNA damage, which in turn reduce your risk of cancer. Their sinigrin content, in particular, has shown to prevent colon cancer. Even though they are one of the most hated vegetables, they contain high concentrations of vitamins A/C and beta carotene.

Carrot: Originally carrots were purple, red, white, and yellow in color. In the sixteenth century crossbreeding created their current orange strain. Carrots contain a high level of beta carotene (as you probably already know), plus they have ample traces of Vitamins B/C/D/E/G/K. They strengthen teeth, improve eyesight, and reduce the risk of infection. In Europe carrot juice is often used to aid in the recovery of those suffering from many cancers and ulcers. Those with eczema have reported that mixing carrot juice with a little salt has been a beneficial natural treatment. Best of all you don't need a doctor's note to buy carrots.

Did You Know: *Hippocrates believed that if a woman consumed carrot seeds she could reduce her risk of pregnancy. Modern science is starting to suggest this may be true by blocking progesterone synthesis.*

Cabbage: Cabbage is loaded with Vitamin U. Red cabbages are packed with folate, while green varieties are notorious for their magnese and vitamin B6. All cabbages reduce the risk of estrogen related cancers. Plus a study out of Berkley shows that they may reduce the risk of prostate cancer. We're still learning all of the amazing preventative properties that this vegetable contains. Cabbage juice is a great remedy for ulcers because of its glutamine content. It may also relieve a cough. Just be sure to drink cabbage juice immediately after juicing, since it can lose part of its nutritional value after it sets. Even though cabbages are a typically a little over 90% water, don't let this fool you. They still pack a powerful punch of nutrition. Plus, their selenium content can reduce the effects of aging.

Cauliflower: The plant sterols and phytochemicals in cauliflower can act as an anti-estrogen agent. This can lower the risk of prostate, breast, cervical, and ovarian cancers. Their high vitamin C content is a strong supporter of the immune system. Cauliflower is one of those things that is so easy to integrate into your diet when it's in the house, whether plain, tossed into a salad, or integrated into a recipe.

Celery: The ancient Romans considered celery to be an aphrodisiac. With modern science we now know that celery contains the pheromone androsterone. In the eighteenth century, it was consumed by females to enhance their beauty and males for stamina. Then in 1897, a Sears catalog featured a celery tonic. It is a good source of potassium, fiber, and vitamin C. Best of all, you burn more calories eating it than you consume. A typical stalk of celery contains about 10 calories, and the human body burns way more than that in digestion alone.

Did You Know: *There is a museum devoted to celery in Portage, Michigan.*

Chicory: Chicory is not very popular, but do not let that discourage you. It contains a natural insulin that is beneficial for diabetics. Chicory has been used to treat circulation, inflammation, and digestion issues. It is also considered to be a powerful cleansing agent of the liver and gallbladder. Chicory is a good source of vitamin A, potassium, and calcium. It also has a natural sedative effect. It won't knock you out, but it may help ease the jitters of an energy drink induced zombie coma that many of us are in. Ironically chicory root once served as a coffee replacement in the early 1800s. It is also a known appetite suppressant.

Collard Greens: Collard greens can help fight hemorrhoids, constipation, and even colon cancer. They are an all around booty booster. The di-indolyl-methane in collard greens make them a strong protector against cancer and a great boost for immunity. Juicing these leaves and mixing them with a sweet fruit makes for a phenomenal beverage.

Caution: *Those dealing with thyroid issues and kidney stones should avoid collard greens.*

Corn: While easily dismissed as a summertime cookout delight, corn is actually quite good for you. It contains folate, thiamin, pantothenic acid, and vitamin C. It's also a good source of fiber and antioxidants. In case you've ever wondered, you can also juice the stuff. This is not a very common beverage in the United States, but it often found throughout China. Just remove the kernels from the cob and then extract them through your juicer.

Did You Know: *The ears of corn are always an even number.*

Dandelion: Yes, I am referring to that weed you see growing outside. Long known for their healing properties in Europe, dandelion leaves are often dismissed in the United States today. Even the Native Americans were quite aware of this weed's healing properties. Now I don't advocate that you start plucking them out of your neighbor's lawn and start chowing down. You have to be very careful to not eat leaves that are drenched in pesticides and fertilizers. Even worse yet, don't eat the ones that Fluffy went potty on. Now that I have thoroughly grossed you out, let me sell you back on these little weeds. They are a HUGE, HUGE antioxidant. Incorporate some of these in to your diet and you will be consuming a healthy dose of vitamins A/B6/C/E/K, thiamin, riboflavin, fiber, manganese, iron, and calcium. Dandelions are used to prevent and treat breast and lung cancers. In addition, they contain insulin and are successful in lowering blood sugar levels. It is thought that their anti-viral properties may soon become utilized in the treatment of AIDS and herpes. Finally dandelions can help clear up eczema and acne.

Endive: Endive is also sometimes referred to as escarole. Whatever you call it, this vegetable can help reduce glucose levels and lower bad cholesterol. Endive is also a good source of antioxidants and folic acid.

Fennel: Overall fennel is said to be similar in its nutritional make-up to celery, but with a little more of a kick with respect to its flavor. The ancient Greeks loved it. They believed that the consumption of fennel brought you closer with the gods. They also were well aware of its medicinal qualities. The anethole in fennel, one of its oils, is an anti-inflammatory and cancer preventer. It is used to help expel phlegm congestion from the lung area. Women should especially incorporate fennel in to their diets since it is provides relief from menopause and cramping. Fennel has a licorice undertone, so be careful what you pair it with.

Garlic: Not the best choice for your breath, but very satiating to your body. Garlic contains vitamin A/C, iron, zinc, calcium, copper, tin, potassium, thiamin, selenium, and sulfur. It is also a wonderful source of protein! Garlic juice can dissolve mucous and remove parasites from the body. Consuming an ample amount of garlic will even help ward off the flu.

Ginger: This root provides a great kick to your drink. Plus, it prevents atherosclerosis (the hardening of arteries), lowers cholesterol, and promotes cardiovascular health. It can fend off the common cold while boosting immunity. Ginger is said to be even more effective than Dramamine in fighting off sea-sickness. Feeling gassy? No need to take anything. Have some ginger. Many women juice ginger during pregnancy to help alleviate morning sickness. We often hear of people drinking a ginger ale to settle their stomach. Imagine how much more potent a fresh squeezed ginger root could be than a can of soda.

Jicama: Jicama is low in calories, but high in carbohydrates. It is a good source of fiber, potassium, and vitamin C. This vegetable can help ease the symptoms of multiple sclerosis and asthma.

Kale: Kale is an extremely potent source of antioxidants that everyone should try. Kale's dark green juice may be more appealing to the palate of a more advanced juicer. Kale in juice or raw form can help reduce your risk of cancer and stroke. Plus it is very beneficial to your eyesight due to its high lutein and beta-carotene levels.

Leek: Leeks are highly medicinal. They were praised by both Aristotle and Nero. Studies have shown that because they contain kaempferol, they can significantly lower the odds of contracting ovarian cancer. According to the Nurses' Health Study by up to 40%! In addition they are said to reduce the risk of colon and prostate cancers. Leeks boost immunity while lowering cholesterol.

Lettuce: Try to avoid the typical iceberg which is mostly just water, and go with a romaine that has a more dense consistency and concentration of nutrients. Romaine will also help prevent lung cancer. On a more superficial note, it enhances hair growth and clears up your complexion. Did you know that Caesar erected a statue to lettuce, believing that it healed him of illness? Kind of brings a new perspective to Caesar dressing.

Mustard Greens: Mustard greens have lots of phytonutrients that make them great a source of disease prevention. They are also high in vitamin K, folic acid, and dietary fiber. Mustard greens are said to be beneficial in both fighting off colds and combating depression. Depending on their oil content their flavor can range from relatively mild to spicy.

Okra: Okra pods can help alleviate constipation and eliminate free radicals. Their dietary fiber content makes them an excellent choice for those wanting to lose some extra weight. Pregnant women should especially try to integrate a little okra in to their diet due to the folic acid content.

Onion: Onions are easy to integrate into all sorts of recipes, so it's fairy simply to add them into your diet on a consistent basis. You can even juice them! While not the most appetizing sounding juice, it is extremely good for you. You can mix it with some honey to make it bearable. Onion juice has also been known to promote virility and dislodge mucous. Whether in their whole or juiced form the quercetin housed in onions is a powerful antioxidant. Onions act as an antihistamine, aid in cellular repair, and can help dissolve blood clots. Don't overdo it in one sitting though; too much onion can actually make you sleepy. It is a natural sedative.

Parsnip: Parsnips look like faded carrots. Don't let the diluted color fool you, they are still a powerhouse for your health. This succulent plant has been used for treating kidney disease. It is also recommended for those struggling with obesity and cellulite. According to university studies parsnips may help reduce inflammation and offer protection from colon cancer and leukemia.

Peas: Peas can be argued as the most nutritious legume. They are rich in phytonutrients, as well as folic and ascorbic acid. The consumption of peas can help reduce your risk of stomach cancer.

Potato: Put your fryer back in the cupboard and pull out the juicer. Yes, potato juice. It's a simple sugar for the body to digest. Many love this drink for its ability to help clear up skin blemishes. The most nutritious part of a potato is its skin.

Did You Know: *You should not store onions and potatoes near one another. Their gases will cause them to spoil faster.*

Radish: The ancient Greeks served radishes on golden platters and Confucius wrote about their healing effects nearly 2500 years ago!! Add some radish into your diet to clear up your sinuses, relieve a cough, reduce nausea, dissolve gallstones, or detoxify your body (especially your liver).

Rhubarb: Rhubarb contains one of the least calories of any vegetable. It is enriched with vitamin K, lutein, and calcium. Translation: It's good for your bones, brain health, and neutralizing free-radicals.

Shallot: Opt to replace onions for shallots whenever possible, since they contain more vitamins and antioxidants. You might be pleasantly surprised that they are less pungent and complement other ingredients quite effortlessly. Shallots can also serve as a nice alternative to garlic. Especially since they don't have that same nasty effect on your breath. Shallots contain something called allicin which is beneficial to your vascular health.

Spinach: Any dark green leafy vegetable is good for you and spinach is no exception. Its high iron content makes it a highly beneficial food for those struggling with anemia. Spinach's anti-inflammatory properties make it a fantastic dietary choice for those struggling with asthma, arthritis, and even Alzheimer's. It's even a mild laxative and can help eliminate a stubborn cough. Good for the skin, fights cataracts, and promotes macular health... what a vegetable! Oh, and did I mention it does wonders for your complexion?

Sweet Potato: A sweet potato actually has a higher beta-carotene content than a carrot. They also contain the phytochemicals, quercetin and chlorogenic acid. But that's not all. If you're looking for vitamins B6/C/D, iron, magnesium, and potassium, then sweet potatoes are the way to go. They can alleviate stress and protect against aging. Enjoy a sweet potato juice while contributing to your cardiovascular and eye health.

Swiss Chard: This leafy Mediterranean delight can help fight osteoporosis, anemia, cardiovascular diseases, and many cancers. High in protein, fiber, vitamins, and minerals, while low in calories, this green will make a great addition to your kitchen.

Squash: Smokers should integrate squash into their diets on a consistent basis. Squash decreases the likelihood of lung cancer and emphysema. Plus it alleviates inflammation, decreases the likelihood of birth defects in expectant mothers, and promotes cardiovascular health. This raw food favorite is rich in vitamins A/C, beta-cryptoxanthin, folate, maganese, and magnesium.

Turnip: Turnips are low in calories and have zero fat. Don't worry though, they're loaded with the good stuff: magnesium, folic acid, vitamin C, calcium, phosphorus, lutein, and zeaxanthin. It is said that incorporating this starchy vegetable into your diet on a regular basis will help reduce your chances of cataracts, hypertension, heart problems, and certain cancers, all while boosting your immunity. It is thought that those suffering with asthma can experience some relief by incorporating more turnips into their diets.

Watercress: Yum! Watercress is not just fun to say, but really good for you. Did you know that Hippocrates used to treat his patients with this stuff? In the middle ages, it was considered a cure for baldness and toothaches. So why do we not talk about its medicinal qualities today? Its positive effects have not been debunked. In fact we have more evidence than ever before to believe that we should enjoy this crunchy delight. A study by the University of Minnesota, showed that smokers benefited by excreting more cigarette carcinogens when incorporating a healthy amount of watercress consistently in to their diet. If we broke down it's nutritional value, it would pretty much resemble a multi-vitamin. So you may be wondering, why not just pop a vitamin and forget about it? Because vitamins are best absorbed in to the human body as food. A pill is better than nothing, but not optimal if you want to enjoy all the benefits that vitamins have to offer.

Yam: Often confused with a sweet potato, yams are actually quite different. They have a starchier consistency and are typically drier. Their allantoin can help abscesses and boils. Plus, the presence of decoction in yams helps to stimulate the appetite. Juicing yams yields to a beverage that is good for those experiencing diarrhea, diabetes, or coughing.

Zucchini: See squash.

7 THE REST OF THE RAW PYRAMID

Let's face it...we can't live on fruits and vegetables alone. Okay, well maybe we can, but that would make for some pretty boring mealtimes. We will briefly discuss the other elements contained within the typical raw food pyramid.

Sprouts

Sprouts are like candy in the health food store. I may be exaggerating just a tad, but experimenting with them can be quite fun and scrumptious. I think we all probably remember some elementary school project involving a moist plastic baggy and something that looked like a bean. Then we went off to play some freeze tag, successful outmaneuvered the cooties, and went on with our lives. For many of us the extent of our sprout knowledge, other than seeing alfalfa sprouts in our grocer's refrigerator, stops there. It is most definitely worth your while to become better versed in the world of sprouts during your adult life.

You may be wondering... just what exactly is a sprout? It is a seed, legume, nut, or grain soaked in a small amount of water to germinate. Germination simply means that the seed begins to grow. When you eat a growing sprout it is abundant with nucleic acid. This is what we're talking about when we refer to "living food". The science of sprouting lets you consume something in its prime state of energy. A sprout is packed with vitamins, amino acids, phytochemicals, minerals, and proteins. Its super high antioxidant content will help fight free radicals and keep your immune system in excellent condition. Best of all, sprouts are an alkalizing miracle food that fight aging.

Buying sprouts that are already grown can be quite costly, but growing them yourself is incredibly frugal and will leave you with a large and continuous fresh supply. Overall it takes just a few minutes to grow a batch, and you'll reap your benefits in merely a few days. They don't take much space, cost hardly anything, and are almost impossible to mess up (even for those lacking a green thumb). Do be careful though, since you are dealing with moisture, mold is always a risk. If you notice that there may be mold spores on your sprouts, dispose of them immediately. They're quite inexpensive and it's simply not worth the risk of getting ill. Mold is a rare occurrence, but something you necessarily must remain aware of. Rinsing your sprouts at least three times a day is a good preventative measure.

There are a plethora of sprouting options out there. First, there are beans. Popular options include garbanzo, mung, and lentils. Then there are leafy sprouts such as alfalfa and clover. You can even do nut and seed varieties, like pumpkin or almond. If you are a true raw foodie you will find that the grass varieties will probably appeal to you. Wheatgrass, in particular, is incredibly addicting once you discover its medicinal properties. Some are surprised to learn that even grains can be sprouted. Barley and oats can be consumed in sprout form. If you really want to experiment you can try something a little more exotic, like fenugreek.

Here is a list of some common sprouts, their uses, and benefits...

Alfalfa - The A-lister of sprouts. Enjoy some alfalfa sprouts sprinkled on your salad or sandwich for some sweet flavor and added texture. Alfalfa can help provide protection against certain cancers, osteoporosis, and heart disease.

Barley – This sprout can help increase longevity and stamina as well as boost immunity. Barley sprouts were actually a staple in the diets of Roman gladiators, so that in itself should tell you a little something about their potency. Countries with widespread famine will distribute barley sprouts due to their powerful life sustaining properties.

Broccoli - Throw broccoli sprouts into a salad for their cancer prevention ability. You can also juice these little guys if you prefer. Pulverization will actually help bring out the anti-cancer properties even more. Keep in mind though that their taste is distinct and somewhat strong to a newbie.

Clover - Clover sprouts are unique since they contain an extremely high concentration of isoflavones. They are yet another known cancer preventer. Delicious eaten by themselves or added into your meal for some extra flavor.

Fenugreek – This exotic sprout may help prevent the flu and/or common cold. Overall it's extremely beneficial for any respiratory ailments such as emphysema, bronchitis, sinusitis, and asthma. Fenugreek compliments fruit dishes quite well.

Garbanzo – Garbanzo beans are sometimes referred to as "chickpeas". They are a good source of zinc, fiber, vitamins B6/C, and folate. These sprouts can help with your fiber intake when blended into a hummus.

Lentil - Lentil sprouts are high in protein. They're also excellent in soups (even raw ones).

Mung Bean – Mung beans make for crunchy sprouts which are very popular in Chinese dishes. They are a great source of protein and rather mild in flavor.

Mustard - Add this zingy sprout for some punch to your dish. If you like spicy, then you'll love mustard sprouts. They have a horseradish-like flavor. Mustard sprouts are a good source of protein and antioxidants.

Onion - Pretty much use this sprout in any way that you would typically use an onion itself. Enjoy the benefits of downing a helpful serving of vitamins A/C/D.

Pea - Pea sprouts pair well with a wide variety of other veggies. They contain folate, phosphorous, and potassium.

Radish - Radish sprouts are loaded with vitamins A and C. Plus, they contain quite a bit of calcium. Power up your immunity easily with some radish sprouts sprinkled on top of your salad.

Soybean - Soybean sprouts are high in folate, fiber, and protein. Enjoy them rolled up in a wrap or blended into a sauce.

Sunflower – If you're looking to add some vitamin A/B/E/D, magnesium, potassium, and iron into your diet, sunflower sprouts are your answer. They have a scrumptious nutty aftertaste, but pair well with a variety of foods.

Wheatgrass - Wheatgrass is the food of the gods when it comes to the world of raw. Even a little thimble, as it's often served in juice form (with an orange wedge), will give you a much needed energy boost on a lazy day. People claim that this stuff has cured everything from cancer to depression. It has been also been said to fight anemia, flush out the toxins from the liver, neutralize blood sugar levels, heal a sore throat, improve fertility, numb a toothache, keep hair from turning white, clear up eczema, improve digestion, relieve constipation, improve heart functions, and reduce blood pressure. Plus, its chlorophyll content does wonders for ensuring your bloodstream stays healthy. These are just to name a few of its many claims to fame. If you don't take anything else away from this chapter, I hope you just start to add some wheatgrass into your diet. Your body will thank you for it. If you don't believe me, just try some. You will almost immediately notice how much better you feel.

Your options for integrating sprouts of all kinds, even those not listed here, into your meals are almost endless. You can replace lettuce with sprouts, add them to wraps, steam them with other veggies, eat them raw, grind them into pastes, juice them, and do just about anything else you can think of. I often add sprouts to dishes as a spice. They add flavor and texture to something that might have been otherwise bland. Go to your local health food store and start giving some different varieties a try for yourself.

Legumes

What is a legume? It is any plant that belongs to the Leguminosae family which bears a fruit in the form of a seedpod. These dry seeds are usually high in protein, fiber, iron, and vitamin B. You definitely want to incorporate them into your raw meal plan to prevent the risk of susceptible deficiencies of a diet with little or no meat. They are also often low in fat and contain no cholesterol. Some of the legumes you may be most familiar with include lentils, chick peas, black beans, edamame, lima beans, soy beans, and peas. Legume plants produce more nitrogen than they can use, and farmers can use this to their advantage to enrich the soil of their crops. Often a legume plant's purpose may be something other than consumption, such as being utilized in a dye, perfume, or wood.

When intended for human consumption, legumes are often brought to a boil and simmered in a crockpot. On the raw diet however, we want to try to stay away from heating whenever possible while still being able to enjoy a tasty, healthy, and safe meal. Rawists tend to prepare their legumes by sprouting, soaking, or cooking them at low temperatures. You can sprout your legumes in a mason jar by soaking them and allowing them to then germinate. If you opt to soak, you want to do so for approximately thirty hours depending on the particular legume. Disposing of and replenishing the water content every couple of hours helps to dispose of the toxins. By the time you choose to enjoy your meal they should be soft and edible. Don't forget you can still cook legumes at a low temperature while staying raw. An enjoyable dish in particular is cooking legumes very lightly and then blending them into a hummus.

Nuts & Seeds

If you have eliminated all, or most, meat from your diet you really should begin to incorporate some raw and organic nuts into your routine to ensure that your protein needs are being met. Almonds are an excellent choice. Many rawists like to soak their nuts overnight, either in the fridge or out in the open, and then dehydrate them. Sounds counter-intuitive, but this process can begin sprouting, release some of the potential toxins, and excrete enzyme inhibitors that are hard on your digestive tract. If you are looking to begin the sprouting process it is important to remember that most of the nuts you will buy from the supermarket will likely not be sproutable since they have undergone pasteurization. You will typically have to purchase nuts for sprouting either from a health food store or your local farmer's market. Nuts are high in fat, but not to worry, it is the monounsaturated kind. A fat your body needs and utilizes to keep you healthy. On a completely raw diet nuts and seeds will be one of your main sources of fat.

Seeds are also monounsaturated. Add a handful of pumpkin, sesame, hemp, or sunflower seeds into your diet plan for some vitamin E, zinc, and fiber. Hemp seeds do not need to be germinated and provide an excellent source of protein. Nuts and seeds are not only a staple for raw foodies because of their protein and fat, but also due to their flavor and ability to substitute many dairy products. Blended into recipes nuts and seeds can make meals feel heavier and more substantial.

Grains

With respect to the raw food diet, grains can be tricky. You should not eat most of them raw in their raw form, nor would you want to. You don't normally see someone salivating at the sight of a wheat leaf in a field. This is with due reason. But then again certain type of raw oats can be enjoyed in cereals. Generally speaking though, uncooked oats are not the most popular choice in the world of raw foods. Many don't like the taste and particular oats may not be ideally suited for raw consumption. For example, you wouldn't want to eat raw quinoa. It's simply too hard to digest. But why not cook it at a low temperature and then throw it into your fresh, raw salad. Or maybe enjoy some warm and hearty oatmeal for breakfast with your raw fruit. I find whole grains in their cooked form to be very complimentary to raw food. The combination can make for some comfort food, which many complain that the raw diet in itself lacks.

Grains remain in murky water in raw food territory. Some people love them, especially when we're talking sprouted, while others consider them to be Satan's spawn in food form. Grains are a part of the regular food pyramid and contain fiber and vitamins. Do you really need them to survive? I suppose not. But why eliminate them? Some say that the nutrition you find in grains, you can obtain elsewhere. Others are concerned about gluten and inflammation. Grains are processed by your body like sugar, raise insulin levels, and can cause you to crave more leading to weight gain. So yes, there are some negative factors. But then there are reputable sources out there, such as the Mayo Clinic and the Food & Drug Administration who consider grains to be integral to a healthy diet.

My approach to grains, is like with everything else in your diet... moderation is key. If you enjoy grains, there is no need to give them up. Just know that there are two main types and understand the differences between the two so you are able to make well-informed shopping decisions.

Refined Grains: I have often heard refined grains compared to paste... sticky, heavy, and not exactly a pleasure to digest. Refined grains have endured substantial processing. Parts of their structure, such as the bran and sperm, have been removed to extend sell dates. Basically if you remove the important parts of the grain you don't have to worry about it spoiling. But as a result, the grain contains less nutritional value. Fiber content is stripped during the milling process. Due to the lack of fiber these refined grains cause your blood sugar to spike. Examples of refined grains include white rice and flour. You will sometimes hear refined grains being referred to as the white grains.

Many refined grains are later enriched. What this means is that they have been fortified with some of the nutritional value that they may have lost during the processing phase, typically vitamin B or folate.

Whole Grains: Whole grains are the good guys as their germ, hull, endosperm, and bran are still intact. Overall they are better sources of fiber and nutritional value. Whenever possible opt for a whole grain versus one that is refined. Realistically, the switch is not going to make a huge difference in your overall health, but nutrition is all about the small choices. When you consistently make good decisions, given the plethora of options that exist, only then will you start to notice your body looks and feels different. Examples of whole grains include barley, oatmeal, and brown rice.

Nutritional Yeast

You know that you're starting to get serious about eating right when you start keeping nutritional yeast on hand. Especially when you start playing word association and when someone shouts "Fungus!" you yell "Yum!". Nutritional yeast can be found in either flake or powder form at your local health food store. It's really not as gross as it initially sounds. This yeast is grown on molasses so it really does have a pleasant taste.

While many are deterred from the raw food diet because they are afraid it will be bland, nutritional yeast is a raw vegan option to infuse some bold flavor into your meals. Many describe it as nutty and even cheese-like. Not only is it full of flavor, but loaded with nutritional value.

Overall nutritional yeast is a great source of protein, fiber, and folic acid. It is also enriched with vitamin B12, which is something that many vegans and vegetarians consciously try to add to their diets. While nutritional yeast is generally fortified with B12, this is not always the case, so be sure to check your labels. If you purchase the fortified type, store it in a dark area if possible. Prolonged exposure to light can destroy the B12 content. Nutritional yeast does not contain gluten, sugar, or dairy and is low in both fat and sodium. It's also kosher and not genetically modified.

Do not confuse nutritional yeast for yeast extract, used for bread, or brewer's yeast, used for beer. It does not have any leavening or fermenting power. This yeast is actually a living microorganism, but it is not a raw food since it undergoes pasteurization. This is so that potentially harmful bacteria are eliminated and the yeast thereby becomes inactived. You really never went to consume "live" yeast, it could continue to grow in your body and deprive you of vital nutrients. So while you may not be 100% raw by adding nutritional yeast powder or flakes to your meals, it's an excellent method to keep you healthy and animal free.

Nutritional yeast is quite a versatile condiment. Since it doesn't require refrigeration, you can even take it on the go. It is commonly used to replace cheese in raw recipes. You can add it a top of popcorn, soups, pastas, and anything else you can think of. Some even like to spinkle it into smoothies. It's all about experimentation.

Oils

Anybody who thinks rawists don't enjoy flavor, has a very elementary understanding of just how varied the raw diet can be. They use oil to add taste to their food just like everyone else, but they prefer raw, vegan, organic cold-pressed oils that do not contain trans-fatty acids or hydrogenated fats. Cold-pressed oils offer a lesser yield so they are not popular amongst company's catering to the general public. These companies can get a lot more out of each batch by heating the source of the oil to an extremely high temperature, even though this eliminates some of the oil's nutritional integrity. Cold-pressed oils however are never heated above 115 degrees Fahrenheit. They are made by grinding the ingredient, whether fruit, nut, seed, etc., and turning that ingredient into a paste like substance. Then the oil content is separated out of the consistency.

Here are some examples of some common oils which you can find cold-pressed and raw friendly...

Almond Oil - Almond oil has a rich flavor that can add substance to all kinds of raw foods. Essentially you can use it as a substitute for any recipe that would call for olive oil. It's a monounsaturated fat that can increase the growth of good bacteria in the stomach. A spoonful three or four times a day can have a laxative effect, but this should only ever be done on a very temporary basis, if ever at all.

Coconut Oil - Coconut oil is used as a staple in many parts of the world and with due reason. It is advantageous to your health and can add a fresh flavor to your dish. Coconut oil is not only rich in nutrients, but it's also an antimicrobial. Consumption can decrease bad cholesterol, while raising the good. Whenever possible, opt for virgin coconut oil as it will not be refined, deodorized, or bleached.

Evening Primrose Oil - The small yellow flower that is the source of this oil has been long known for its medicinal properties. One of its unique characteristics is that it contains a high concentration of gamma-linoleic acid which is an anti-inflammatory. In addition it is good for your skin, nails, and hair. Evening primrose is a famed anti-aging substance. Studies have also shown it to be beneficial on a neurological level. Finally it has shown to positively reduce eczema and increase fertility.

Olive Oil – It almost seems insulting to add olive oil to the list amongst all of the other oils, as it's so acclaimed. Those who use olive oil versus any of the other traditional "cooking" or "uncooking" oil out there have a significantly lesser risk of heart disease. Olive oil can help lower bad cholesterol, prevent ulcers, and regulate blood sugar. It's definitely the A-lister of this section, due to its notoriety and healing properties.

Poppy Seed Oil - Poppy seeds were praised by the ancient Greeks as being a source of strength. And those old time Greeks were on to something. Poppy seeds are rich in linoleic acid which is considered beneficial to cardiovascular health. Plus, their oleic acid may help prevent against breast cancer. This smooth oil makes a phenomenal choice for salad dressings. An interesting thing to note is that raw friendly varieties have more kick to their flavor than the traditional ones. They are less processed and retain more of the natural poppy flavor.

Sesame Seed Oil - Centuries ago the Assyrians considered sesame seed oil to be medicinal. It was generally confined to the wealthiest citizens due to its limited supply. This oil has long been used to relieve stress. It's extremely high in antioxidants and does wonders for the skin.

Sunflower Oil – This pressed oil from sunflower seeds is polyunsaturated and heart healthy. It is low in saturated fat and contains no trans fat whatsoever. Sunflower oil is high in vitamin E, phytochemicals, and antioxidants. It's a very versatile oil that especially adds a wonderful taste to nori and salads. While I certainly don't recommend frying, if you must, sunflower oil is the way to go.

Some rawists are against the use of oils altogether. They may contend that the amount of fat is simply not worth the caloric content. Others will argue that their consumption is highly advantageous and serves as a catalyst for the absorption of nutrients that your body desperately needs. I happen to agree with the latter group. Regardless of whether oils aid in absorption, it seems silly to make an argument against oils for their calories. The raw diet is typically low in caloric intake, especially when compared to the Standard American Diet, so it's rather irrelevant. This moot point hardly seems worth skimping out on the added flavor and nutritional benefits.

Seaweed

Before you make a face of disgust imagining chewing on a hunk of slimy grass, give seaweed a fair chance. If you think about it, what's the difference between ocean grown plants and the thousands that grow on dry land, besides saltiness and texture? The only notable distinction is seaweed's vastly superior nutritional composition.

Seaweeds, also known as marine algae, are ancient plants that have been consumed by the Japanese as early as 300 BC. They are still regularly consumed in Japan, Korea, and China. Regions in the Caribbean take advantage of seaweed's medicinal properties and utilize them as an elixir to remedy common ailments. It somewhat surprises me that they haven't caught on as more of a staple in the diets of Americans. But then again, McSeaweed doesn't really have that great of a ring to it.

I will say, however, that within the smaller niche populations of nutrition oriented communities and pop culture magazines, seaweed is gaining quite a bit of attention. It's still rather dormant nonetheless, when compared to its utilization in other parts of the world. Sure it's used in sushi, but that's about the only time we see seaweed come in contact with our plates here in the United States.

There are literally thousands of different types, as there are with land plants. Not all seaweeds are edible, but a good cluster of them make for a fine meal. Some of the specific seaweed varieties that are used for human consumption are farmed and their cultivation has developed into quite an industry. The most popular types enjoyed by connoisseurs include... nori, kelp, arame, irish moss, kombu, and wakame.

Seaweeds are usually broken down and categorized based on their coloration. Strains include green, red, and brown.

Green (Chlorophyta) - This type of seaweed thrives in a marine or freshwater environment. There are three subcategories: unicellular, multicellular, and colonial. Green seaweeds make for excellent salads. Plus they will fight anemia and impotence all while providing a boost to your metabolism and memory. Their beta carotene content may also be beneficial in cancer treatment. Green varieties serve as an important food source to oceanic life and can be found in many cosmetic products.

Red (Rhodophyta) - While we say red, this may also include seaweed that has a purplish hue. This group of oceanic life may be beneficial for osteoporosis, heart disease, dementia, and diabetes.

Many crustaceans and fish thrive on this type of seaweed for nourishment; especially since it can survive at incredible depths of the ocean floor. Popular varieties include Irish moss and nori.

Brown (Phaeophyta) - Brown seaweeds are found everywhere from the Tropics to the Arctic. According to researchers at the University of Newcastle brown seaweed can protect the lining of your stomach and provide you with an extended amount of energy while helping you feel satiated. Research from Kyoto University gives us reason to believe that brown seaweed has the ability to improve cardiovascular health, reduce the risk of stroke, and even lower blood pressure. A famous type of seaweed of this category is kelp.

The benefits of seaweed are plentiful. Within the plant itself, powerful antioxidants are stored. It's a great choice for detoxification, whether ingested or used as a body wrap. If consumed, seaweed can help alkalize your body while providing you with much nourishment. Unlike land which is over-farmed and where nutrients are often depleted from our food's soil, the sea is abundant with rich nutrients. Sure there are now seaweed farms, but these are, relatively speaking, a more recent phenomenon. Seaweed may just provide the largest variety of minerals in a single food that is readily available for human consumption. Interestingly enough the makeup of the nutrients in seaweed are rather similar in composition to hemoglobin.

Seaweed has been known to aid in thyroidal healing. It is the world's richest source of pure iodine in a food. Accordingly, a study from the Canadian University, McGill, found that there is evidence to support seaweed aiding detoxification from nuclear radioactivity. A senior research scientist at Greenpeace claimed that seaweed had a similar effect in removing the toxins of lead and cadmium that are often found in cigarette smoke.

Dr. Jane Teas of Harvard University published a piece suggesting that the increased rates of seaweed consumption in Japan, versus other parts of the globe, may help account for the low rates of breast cancer there. This can be explained by the lignans which are found in seaweed since they are known to inhibit estrogen synthesis on a cellular level. The folate content of seaweed may also prevent colon cancer. Is this stuff amazing or what? And there's still more!

Teacher, Greg Lampert, of the College of Integrated Chinese Medicine believes that kelp has the ability to reduce phlegm and swelling.

Seaweed is also an excellent option for those looking to enhance their complexion and the luster of their hair. Whenever you are feeling stressed, consuming some seaweed can have a calming effect since it contains magnesium and pantothenic acid. If seaweed is powerful enough to help generate electricity imagine what it can do for your body.

It may all sound too good to be true, and perhaps it is. But so far what we know about seaweed seems to be very promising. There are a few risks. You may want to opt for organic varieties, since regular seaweed may contain traces of arsenic. It also has a heap of sodium per serving so you will want to regulate your consumption.

Adding a tad of seaweed into your raw food diet is rather simple. You can integrate it into salad, soup, green juice, sushi, or dressing seamlessly. You can also dehydrate it for a crunchier texture. You can even find seaweed flakes to sprinkle a top of your food, if that's more your thing. However you choose to do it, try to add some seaweed into your diet in some manner. It's well worth it!

Microalgae

While seaweeds fall under the classification of macroalgae there are smaller types of algae that grow on a microscopic level which are referred to as microalgae. When it comes to food I'm always an advocate of keeping it simple. Well, why not opt for the simplest life form of all? I mean, if it's gotten us this far.

These tiny ancient life forms do not have stems, roots, or leaves but still play a vital role in the bottom of the food chain even today. Some speculate that the manna of the Bible may have actually been dried spirulina. Even though this food was popular in times long ago, we're still learning of its nutritional benefits to this day. Microalgae can be used as a bio-fuel and its new potential benefits to our diet are still being discovered.

Hundreds of thousands of varieties are known to exist. Some of these types are edible and rawists are cashing in on the many benefits. Spirulina and chlorella are the two most common nutritional microalgae supplements. Spirulina is known to have been a food source to the Aztecs and may have possibly been used by even earlier civilizations. It's a blue-green algae that flourishes in warm waters. Spirulina is packed with gamma linolenic acid, beta-carotene, maganese, zinc, selenium, copper, iron, and vitamins B and E. It's rather amazing that something so teeny can contain so many vitamins, antioxidants, and minerals. One of the main reasons that spirulina is so favored by the raw population is because of its high protein content. Up to three times that of meat!

If you think that it's loaded with lots of good stuff, just wait until you hear all that it can do for you. It can act as an antihistamine for allergy sufferers. Plus it may promote liver health and fight against oral cancers. It was approved in Russia to help eliminate the effects of exposure to radioactivity, since it helps to supercharge immunity. Lab studies have even shown spirulina to counter herpes infections in animals. Whether this is true for the human population, we still do not know.

The second microalgae worth discussing is chlorella. While not that popular in mainstream America today, these microscopic algae received a lot of attention around early to mid twentieth century. They were thought of as a potential food source to combat world hunger. Especially, since they were such an abundant source of protein and vitamins. Chlorella never really lived up to its humanitarian potential though. It never even beat its top competitor, spirulina. It does however remain a popular food choice for those who enjoy maintaining optimal dietary health.

Chlorella has the ability to eliminate metallic toxins from the body, such as mercury. It can enhance immunity and even eliminate body odor. Chlorella is said to be helpful in dealing with cancers, hypoglycemia, asthma, and depression. Its magnesium content is also wonderful for cardiovascular health. And it can lower blood pressure. Who would think that pond scum could do all that?

I predict that in coming years we will see a rise in the popularity and consumption of microalgae as a food source. It rather stuns me that it is not more heavily integrated into the diet of Americans today. Especially when you consider how potent and powerful these sources of vitality can be. Just a little bit goes a very long way.

Herbs & Spices

Just because we like our food raw, doesn't mean we prefer it to be bland. Flavor can, and should, be a big part of why you enjoy a raw food diet. There are two simple ways to add some taste to a dish, herbs and spices. Often people use the words interchangeably and refer to a dried herb as a spice and vice versa. Both have similar uses and potential medicinal properties.

Herbs: Herbs come from the leaves of plants. You can use a liberal amount of them in your cooking (or as we say here, uncooking) to add flavor to your dishes. Herbs have long been utilized for their medicinal properties.

Spices: Spices come from the root, flower, bark, or seed of a plant. You generally don't want to add much of a spice to a dish as they can be very overwhelming. Spices are also known for their preservation abilities.

In ancient times, both of these flavorings, especially spices, were prized possessions. A luxury only afforded by the rich. Today we all have access to these delights and can grow many in the comfort of our own homes or purchase them for a reasonable price at the supermarket.

When it comes to herbs you always want to go as fresh as possible. Optimally grow them yourself on a windowsill. It's an amazing feeling to grow and eat your own food. Besides being very cost conscious. By opting for a fresh version of an herb, rather than its dried counterpart, you will be enjoying a greater amount of the available nutrients.

I hear a lot of raw food experts talk about the dangers of these flavorings. Just go online and search "natural hygiene" and you'll find a wide array of herb haters out there. I'm not saying they're wrong. I'm just saying that to the best of my knowledge herbs and spices really aren't that big of a threat to humanity. They are not a poison in normal doses. And if they can positively contribute to the taste of your meal, so you can eat more of those healthy things that your body needs, then by all means, sprinkle away. Yes, herbs and spices in massive quantities, more than any rational human being would consume in one sitting, can be toxic. Common sense would tell you that too much of any food is a bad thing. There's a reason too much seasoning on your dish tastes disgusting. Herbs and spices in normal quantities, however, can be quite beneficial.

There are many holistic healing advocates out there who believe that herbs and spices are actually gems to be uncovered. "Ayurveda" is a word you may hear thrown around at your favorite spa, but you may not know exactly what it is and how it relates to the flavorings in your dishes. Ayurveda is Sanskrit for the science of life. It is holistic therapy that creates perfect harmony for both the body and mind. Ayurveda is preoccupied with prevention, while the western world tends to focus on healing ailments after they occur. Just imagine how much simpler it is to maintain health than to try to regain it. An aryuvedic philosophy suggests that herbs and spices have medicinal properties and should be incorporated into our diets to promote overall health and well-being. Modern research confirms that the antioxidant, anti-microbial, and anti-viral properties of herbs and spices make them quite beneficial.

You just have to know what types of herbs and spices to use and how to incorporate them into your diet. You can use them to enhance your food or even to create a tea beverage. Here is a list of some common herbs and spices along with their benefits...

Allspice - Allspice can help relieve indigestion and flatulence while regulating blood sugar. It is an antiseptic and anesthetic. Allspice makes a wonderful additive to both soups and sweets.

Anise - With a licorice-like flavor this spice can help relieve the common flu or cold. Those suffering with asthma find it to be extremely beneficial. Anise easily compliments both sweet and savory dishes.

Basil - This seasoning is quite popular in Mediterranean cuisine. It's an anti-inflammatory and suspected to reduce cholesterol levels.

Bay Leaves - Another Mediterranean favorite. Bay leaves can help prevent weight gain and regulate blood sugar levels. However I do not recommend that you enjoy bay leaves in their raw form. They present a choking hazard and do not easily digest. I have heard of fellow rawists blending them, but proceed with caution.

Black Pepper – While one of the most common spices in our cooking today, it's not really all that good for you. It's not harmful, just not worth bragging about. Black pepper is said to calm flatulence and an upset stomach.

Capers – Adored by Mediterranean chefs, capers play a leading role in tartare and many salads. They are an appetite stimulant which aid digestion.

Caraway - This is a spice you may not have heard of, but you're probably familiar with its flavor. It's what makes sauerkraut and rye bread taste distinct. Caraway is thought to prevent aging, neurological damage, cancer, and infection.

Cardamom – Cardamom can help alleviate heartburn. Excellent used in chai and sweets.

Cayenne Pepper - Popular in Thai and Mexican dishes, cayenne pepper can help increase blood flow, fight infection, enhance memory, and regulate metabolism.

Celery Seed - Celery seed is popular in Mediterranean cuisine. This additive can aid an upset stomach and relieve gas. It also has a calming effect on nervousness and can ease a stress related headache.

Chervil - Also known as "fancy parsley". It is rather mild in taste but medicinally potent in its ability to purify the blood.

Cilantro - Cilantro is a member of the carrot family. It is used to treat nausea, inflammation, stress, gas, headaches, coughs, and urinary tract infections. This plant can also help aid digestion. Like microalgae, it can also help remove metals from the body. Cilantro is popular amongst the raw population especially since it is best consumed in its raw form. People tend to have a strong love or hate relationship with cilantro's distinct flavor.

Cinnamon - This spice may lower blood sugar and as little as a half teaspoon a day has shown to lower LDL cholesterol. A recent study out of Maryland showed that cinnamon had the ability to inhibit the proliferation of leukemia and lymphoma. Another study at the University of Copenhagen found that patients suffering from arthritis showed major improvements when adding a mixture of honey and cinnamon to their breakfast. Cinnamon is also thought to be a great memory booster. Who would have thought that your Cinnamon Dolce latte could help you ace that next exam? Additional benefits of cinnamon include stress relief and the ability to fend off the common cold. The essential oil found within cinnamon, euganol, is an anesthetic and antiseptic which has shown to lower blood sugar.

Cloves - Prized in Indian dishes, cloves are used to treat a toothache, upset stomach, and provide relief from congestion. Be careful though, cloves in large doses can be toxic. But I really cannot say that I have ever met anyone who enjoys sitting home on a Saturday night chomping on heaping spoonfuls of cloves. Just don't tack on clove leaves as a new section to your food pyramid and you should be alright.

Coriander – See cilantro.

Cumin - Cumin is the second most popular spice in the world. Pepper being the first. Cumin is somewhat pungent and also used to treat an upset stomach. It is also said to be great for memory.

Curry - This Indian delight is actually a blend of various spices, including turmeric. While it can fight cancer, curry powder may affect your body's ability to clot blood. Do not ingest curry anytime you are about to go in for surgery.

Dill - Rather sweet in flavor, dill is an excellent mild addition to many dishes, especially salad dressing or vegetable dip. Dill can help relieve nervousness and headaches.

Epazote – This Latin American favorite can help provide relief from indigestion, cramps, and even ulcers.

Fennel - Anise-like in taste, fennel can relieve inflammation and improve digestion. It's a favorite in Italian cooking. Fennel is a wonderful natural agent in relieving congestion.

Garlic - Garlic can be added to just about everything, except sweets. It can help boost your immunity and help maintain normal blood pressure and cholesterol levels. Ancient traditions used garlic to treat a cough.

Ginger - Sweet and peppery this commonly used Asian food additive can help settle an uneasy stomach. It is also an anti-inflammatory and may help relieve pain.

Lemongrass – Popular in tea form, this herb alleviates stress, eliminates headaches, and can help clear up the common infections to blame for a sore throat.

Marjoram - Marjoram is the long lost cousin of mint and oregano. In the Mediterranean it is often enjoyed as a tea. Medicinally marjoram may help prevent muscle spasms.

Mint - Mint can help soothe a troubled tummy and is a common remedy for those who struggle with Irritable Bowel Syndrome. It's antiviral and antimicrobial. Peppermint is now being studied for providing potential pain relief, especially to the stomach region. The spearmint variety is mostly enjoyed for its flavor, rather than its medicinal properties. Nevertheless, it is beneficial for respiratory related elements.

Mustard Seed - Full of omega-3s, calcium, fiber, iron, zinc, manganese, magnesium, phosphorus, protein, and selenium, it's no surprise that mustard seeds are good for you. They can give your metabolism a boost, while relieving muscle pain. When mustard oil is applied to your scalp it can stimulate hair growth.

Nutmeg - Nutmeg is notorious as a Christmas delight. It comes from an evergreen tree. Not so much a Christmas tree, but rather its tropical variety. It's a great addition to both sweets and sauces. Nutmeg has often been used to treat congestion. Something interesting that you might not have known about nutmeg is that it's actually a mild hallucinogen.

Onion Powder – Onion powder added to your meal can help you sweat out a cold. Just don't share your meal with Fido, onion powder is toxic to dogs.

Oregano - If you've ever eaten Greek food, you are familiar with oregano. It's a distinct bitter spice that is very high in antioxidants and contains Omega-3 fatty acids, potassium, vitamins A/C, iron, niacin, copper, manganese, boron, and fiber. It can stimulate immunity and help prevent heart disease. Oregano has antibacterial and antifungal properties.

Paprika – The flavor of paprika greatly varies depending on its origin. This spice is often used in dishes to give them a distinct color. It contains a plentiful amount of vitamin C and capsaicin. Paprika can help your body absorb iron, neutralize stomach acid, and improve blood circulation.

Parsley: Enjoy a few sprigs to freshen your breath, detox your body, and improve your overall energy. In fact, parsley is considered the energy drink of juicers. It has one of the highest chlorophyll contents of any vegetable. Besides, parsley contains a higher level of vitamin C than oranges, and a greater amount of iron than spinach.

Did You Know: *The ancients often utilized parsley for healing cuts, since it is able to draw out puss and reduce the risk of infection.*

Poppy Seeds - Poppy seeds reduce the body's ability to absorb calcium, but this isn't necessarily a bad thing. It may lessen the likelihood of kidney stone development. The poppy plant contains opium alkaloids. Therefore you should avoid eating a poppy seed muffin if you are going in for a blood test the next day. Poppy seeds can make you falsely test positive for drugs. Consuming large quantities of poppy seeds may in fact lead to hallucinations.

Rosemary - Rosemary is an anti-inflammatory and antiseptic with a pine-like flavor. We have found literature that dates back to 1529, prescribing rosemary to those suffering from memory loss. Its carnosic acid is thought to slow Alzheimer's disease. Studies have shown that even just the smell of rosemary can provide a boost to memory. Rosemary is also a natural antidepressant.

Saffron - Saffron is the liquid gold of the cooking world. It is rich in many vitamins and minerals (and price). The safranal oil and alfa-crocin found within the spice are antidepressants and can help fight cancer.

Sage - This peppery evergreen spice can prevent excessive sweating, fight bacterial infections, and regulate blood sugar. Sprinkle sage onto fat and oily foods to ease digestion.

Savory - There are two common types of savories out there, summer and winter blends. They are both herbal mixtures known to relieve a sore throat. Preference is a matter of taste.

Sea Salt – The only difference between sea salt and the regular old table kind is that it contains slightly more minerals; but not enough to really make that big of an impact on your overall health. Sea salt is one of those perpetuated health food myths. It's something triumphantly touted by fast food giants feigning the appearance of concern for their customer's health. Sure it's preferable, but it's no superfood. Simply choose it because it tastes better, not for what it will do for you. Technically, sea salt is neither an herb nor a spice, it's a mineral.

Sesame Seeds – Integrating sesame seeds into your confections, sauces, entrees, etc. can help elevate your mood, support your immune system, and aid in red blood cell production. Sesame seeds also contain anti-cancer properties due to their concentration of lignans. Their nutritional absorption is enhanced in pulverized form.

Stevia – The sweetener of the health food world is actually an herb. While a newfound buzz to pop culture, this sweeter has been utilized regularly for centuries. It is used to aid weight loss, reduce inflammation, lower cholesterol, stabilize blood pressure, and counter depression.

Tamarind – This South American delight is loaded with vitamins. It has a laxative effect and can help remedy bile related disorders.

Tarragon - Terragon has been used to treat insomnia and increase appetite. Scientific studies suggest it may even lower blood sugar levels. It makes a great addition to most salad dressings.

Thyme - Thyme can help relieve cramps and muscle spasms. It also has the power to kill MRSA (Staph) infections. It's excellent sprinkled on vegetables. Did you know that it is also often the main active ingredient, thymol, in mouthwash?

Turmeric - This is a robust seasoning that can be added to give a little punch to your vegetables. It is, in many parts of the world, used as an antiseptic for cuts. Studies on mice show that it even has the ability to kill cancerous cells. Turmeric has even shown to slow the effects of multiple sclerosis on mice. It may also slow the progression of the plaque buildup that leads to Alzheimer's in the human brain. On a more superficial note, turmeric can promote the healing of skin and promote anti-aging in humans. With all of its wonderful health benefits it's no surprise that this spice makes a wonderful tea in Okinawa, Japan. Some Ayurvedic medicine advocates suggest using turmeric as one of the main ingredients in an alternative form of holistic birth control.

Vanilla - The extract from vanilla pods is actually the second most expensive spice after saffron. Vanilla contains traces of many minerals and iron. It is also known to be an aphrodisiac. The vanillin content in vanilla is a powerful antioxidant which may have cancer fighting abilities. In the way we traditionally use vanilla, as a small amount of extract in some desserts, there are really not a lot of benefits to be gained. Just enjoy its sweet aromatic flavor.

Supplements

As discussed in Chapter 1, those eating a predominantly raw diet need to carefully monitor their nutritional intake so that they do not become deficient of the things their body's need. The more we limit that which we consume, the greater the need for concern. Even the healthiest of diets run the risk of deficiencies.

The good news is that it is entirely possible to obtain all of the things your body requires while staying vegan and raw. It just takes more effort. Ensure that you are consuming enough vitamin B12, iron, calcium, and protein. An easy way to make certain of it is to take a supplement of some sort. Supplements can help fill in the gaps where your diet may be lacking.

Final Words

There are endless ways to keep your raw food diet varied and interesting. You just have to be open-minded to trying new things. By incorporating a wide array of foods/supplements into your meals, you can ensure that all of your nutritional needs are being met.

8 THE RAW CARNIVORE

Many who are intrigued by the raw lifestyle find it appealing due to its vegan element. However there are a fair amount of rawists out there who enjoy the delicacies of raw meat and seafood. In fact, one of the most shocking discoveries I made in my research, was finding out just how many people live on a diet that includes raw meat regularly. I had no idea!! I read hundreds of self-written accounts of people who credit raw meat to their good health. I was nothing short of stunned. It simply seems to go against everything we are taught from the time we are children.

I feel it is important to discuss raw meats because they are often given a bad reputation. Much of what we hear is uninformed and unfounded. But then again, the opposite remains true; many don't realize the potential dangers. There is a lack of reputable information out there. Those who go raw and vegan do not bother to investigate raw meat, and logically so, it's not much of a concern for them. While those who do enjoy meat, usually do so cooked. They have never even considered eat it any other way. Logically it makes sense that neither of these groups would be all too concerned about raw meats and only hear tales from the periphery.

Most of us in the United States love to eat meat, and do so regularly, but would find the idea of eating it raw barbaric and grotesque. In many nations raw delicacies are a healthy part of one's diet. Middle Easterners and Inuits incorporate a regular amount of raw meat and fish into their normal diets. Asian cultures have a vast array of scrumptious raw fish dishes. So why in the United States do so many of us consider raw animals to be disgusting? I think some of it has to do with fear of the unknown. It may be foreign and look different. The texture is unlike anything we are familiar with eating.

Another issue is that American teens living in urban areas are rather sheltered. They have little conception of slaughterhouses and hardly associate their meat coming from an animal. Meat in its raw form may present a little less disconnect to these folks. The realization may frighten them. I find that many of those I know, even in their twenties, have never handled raw meat. They live as omnivores on take-out and boxed meals, never having much of a need to cook regularly (or even at all). I suspect that people would be a lot less grossed out by handling a chicken carcass, if they were exposed to the contents of their McNuggets. It's kind of scary how little so many people know about the food they are eating. Raw meat can be shocking to people at first due to lack of exposure and experience. It suddenly seems like a dead animal is lying on their plate for the first time. Eventually one gets over that initial shock and realizes one of two things. One, being that they love it. The other, that they are extremely repulsed (either by the texture, taste, or idea).

There is a greater risk of disease with raw meat, than its cooked counterpart. This is true. But there are certain meats out there that are specifically sold with the intention that they will be consumed raw and are less likely to contain disease carrying pathogens. Raw seafood is relatively less risky, than meat, as the salt water and storage temperatures reduce the risk of bacteria and parasites. Children, seniors, expectant mothers, and those who have a weakened immune system should avoid ingesting raw meat and seafood altogether.

Raw meat always contains an element of risk. Then again, so does getting in your car and going to work every day. The question is, just how dangerous is it? When I first began studying the consumption of raw meat I was dumbfounded at the lack of objective information out there on the subject. I came across tons of personal testimonies of people eating raw carcasses consistently. Then I found more authoritative research, and it terrified me half to death. It sounded like an eminent death sentence, but much more cruel. As though you might as well wash down your tartare with a nice cool glass of arsenic.

I don't prescribe to the philosophies of either of these schools. I'm more of a neutral in this area. A Switzerland of carpaccio, if you will. Basically I remain on the fence on whether I want to advocate it or not. Personally, I do enjoy a steak tartare or carpaccio on occasion and raw fish on a weekly basis. I have never experienced any complications as a result thereof. However I am extremely picky in my selection of dining establishments and never enjoy these things at home (with the exception of pickled herring from my local market). I only eat raw animal products from very reputable restaurants that are notorious for their quality and care. Often this means paying a little more for my food, but I gladly do so for the added comfort of trusting that it is of high quality, fresh, and being handled with care. Even though I do so, I often wonder if I am making a wise decision. Would I advise someone else to do the same? Or is this my little dinner game of Russian roulette?

It is important to be selective about where your meat originates. Is it a quality source that you can trust? Have they ensured that the proper safety measures have been followed? It is important to deep freeze raw meat before consumption to kill potential parasites. Either extreme heat or cold, both, work to eliminate some of the health risks. According to the USDA, cooking foods at a temperature above 150 degrees Fahrenheit breaks down bacteria and prevents it from reproducing. Deep freezing methods will do the same, but not as effectively as heating. Deep freezing will, like heating, unfortunately also kill some of the enzymes, but seems to be considered allowable by the standards of most rawists. Deep freezing should not be confused with simply putting meat in your home freezer. Once you pull the meat out of your residential freezer the bacteria will come back to life and multiply rapidly causing even a greater amount of potential harm than before. This will not be a sufficiently cool enough temperature to kill the bacteria. Temperature is a very crucial element of raw meat consumption.

Raw Ground Beef

Another thing to consider is the type of meat you are eating. Hamburger meat from your grocery store should never be eaten raw. It poses an extremely high risk of illness due to the way it is processed and handled. Therefore you should always eat in its cooked form. Did you know that a single fast food hamburger usually contains between forty to one-hundred different animals? Another issue is over-frugality. In an attempt to scrape every last piece of meat from the cow, you will often find that a tool called an Advanced Meat Recovery Machine is utilized. It is usually to blame for the bone marrow and spinal cord mixed into your ground beef. What a wonderful carrier of Mad Cow Disease! Fast-food restaurants are a little more cautious about tracing the origin of their meats and avoiding the use of Advanced Meat Recovery Machines. In that regard, you would probably be safer eating a cooked hamburger from a major fast-food joint than you would from your local grocery store.

Do not fret that you can never enjoy a cooked hamburger again; you just have to be cautious in your buying choices. According to a study from Cornell University, grass fed cattle pose a lesser risk than those that are grain and by-product fed. Plus the pH levels of the cattle fed corn are similar to that of humans. Therefore the E. Coli that could survive in the cattle, could very well survive in you. Grass fed cows are exposed to fewer pathogens and are raised in open fields. They contain a greater amount of Omega-3 fatty acids and beta carotene due to their diets. Basically if given the option, opt for grass fed cattle whenever possible.

Raw Poultry

Another food you especially want to avoid raw, chicken. There is nothing innately wrong with the chicken itself. In fact, many Japanese restaurants serve a chicken sashimi. The problem lies with our industrial food standards. Chickens are not usually handled with the best care or in a manner that would ensure the safety of them being consumed raw. Besides, they are often fed ground up slaughterhouse remnants and swept up food droppings which are contaminated with waste. Even if they happened to be raised cautiously and handled properly, most people would not find the squeamish raw texture that appetizing. Therefore avoiding raw chicken really doesn't come as that great of a disappointment. I look forward to potentially enjoying some chicken sashimi when visiting Japan, where this meal is commonplace, but would never consider trying it in the States.

Meat Irradiation

Our bodies have a natural defense system that is equipped to handle a certain amount of bacteria just fine. We encounter a greater risk of problems when we have a weakened immunity and/or encounter a piece of food with an increased bacteria content. Many foods, including meats, are now being irradiated to kill this harmful bacteria before they even reach our supermarket shelves. The FDA considers it to be completely safe. It is likened to pasteurizing milk. All irradiated food is required to possess a Radura logo. Keep in mind though; you would never know if the restaurant you are dining in is serving irradiated meat. Due to the stigma, there has been talk the term "irradiated" may soon be replaced with electronically or cold pasteurized.

Overall it seems like irradiating meat does make it safer, which is fantastic and should be a major plus to carnivores out there. But there is a downside. Despite the claims by the FDA, there is speculation on whether or not these irradiated foods are actually safe for human consumption? Next, there are concerns whether any important enzymes or vitamins are lost in the process. Finally, irradiating food is a great excuse to perpetuate lax farming standards. Instead of focusing on the added costs of prevention, ill animals can simply be irradiated and passed along to consumers.

Foodborne Illness

Even though there are precautions that you can take to help reduce the risk of foodborne illness, there is always a greater risk in consuming a raw meat dish than one that is cooked. Personally I consider it a "forbidden delight". I am aware that it's probably not a good idea to consume it too often because of the risk incurred, but I find it to be such a delicacy when prepared the right way. Understand that food poisoning is incredibly likely when purchasing meat from your local grocery store and consuming it raw. You only want to order these types of dishes from restaurants who specialize in raw meat purchasing and preparation.

If you are looking to enjoy some steak tartare, you want to make sure that the cattle were raised in a healthy manner and in a sanitary environment. Only eat raw meat where you trust its origin and handling. You may wonder why this dish is considered safe in so many fine dining restaurants. The reason lies that it is made of filet mignon, which if not cross-contaminated with any other cuts, is relatively safe to eat.

Most meat prepared for human consumption is assumed to be cooked and treated accordingly. Precautions are not taken on a mainstream level to ensure the highest standards of safety. Slaughterhouses may pump cows full of hormones and antibiotics and the increase of grain prices have left many slaughterhouses simply feeding their animals with waste products. These are not things you want to carelessly be dumping into your body. Negligent processing and atrocious conditions can end up leaving disgusting fecal matter all over cattle. How comfortable are you with eating irradiated fecal matter? Personally, I don't care if it the FDA claims it is safe. Irradiated poop is nothing more than disgusting.

As an added precaution against the bacteria content, try an alcohol based sauce. It acts as a disinfectant. Will it eliminate all risk? No. But every little bit helps. It's kind of like wearing your seat belt in a car accident. Will it ensure safety? Not necessarily. But it may help if a crisis strikes.

The following health risks are notoriously incurred from consuming raw meat:

Listeria - Deli meats and unpasteurized milk are the most common contaminated sources. Listeria often goes away on its own, or with the aid of some antibiotics, but it can be incredibly dangerous for those with a weakened immune system.

Salmonella - Unfortunately salmonella is fairly common. Thankfully it goes away on its own within a few days. You'll probably feel terrible, but not suffer from long-term repercussions.

Tapeworms - Raw pork and beef (or even water) can potentially contain a tapeworm. These hideous little creatures can attach themselves to your intestinal wall. Even worse than a tapeworm, are tapeworm eggs which can work their way outside of the intestine and into other vital parts of your body. A tapeworm can live up to twenty years!!

Toxoplasmosis - Eating raw lamb, pork, or beef can lead to this infection with flu-like symptoms. Many healthy people do not require treatment.

Trichinosis - This nasty little disease usually stems from consuming raw (or undercooked) pork, which had previously consumed diseased feed (typically another pig or rodent). After consumption larvae can enter your system and then molt finding their way into your bloodstream.

Regardless of your body's natural ability to fight things off, always consult with your physician immediately if you suspect you've incurred food poisoning. With all of these scary threats it seems ridiculous that anyone would even consider eating raw meat. Now that I've thoroughly freaked you out, let's look at some of the positive factors...

Vitamin B6 - So many of us are presently vitamin B6 deficient. The reason being is that our food is either pasteurized or cooked to kill any harmful bacteria. When we kill the bad elements, we are also killing some of the good. B6 deficiencies are linked with all kinds of dangers, such as cancers, diabetes, heart disease, kidney failure, sickle cell anemia, asthma, carpal tunnel, as well as many other diseases. Vitamin B6 is critical to our general health.

Simplified Digestion – Just as with the other foods we discussed earlier, cooked meats are difficult for your body to digest. By eating enzyme enriched foods, such as those which are raw, we preserve our own enzymes and are able digest much more easily.

Taste - Some people find it incredibly delicious. I can truly say there is nothing like it. Personally I hardly eat any cooked meat. I simply do not find it appetizing. However, in its raw state it's quite a delicacy.

Fertility - There was a notorious study performed by Francis Pottenger, starting in 1932. He observed the health of nine-hundred cats over a decade. The cats were divided into two groups. Half of his cats consumed only raw foods, and the other half only cooked. The raw group showed several signs of greater health and better fertility. According to writings of Dr. Weston Price, in another study observing the Eskimo population, he found that pregnant females who ate a steady diet of raw meats, endured very easy pregnancies with uncomplicated deliveries compared to their modern diet counterparts.

Even though I mention these two studies, I have a major problem considering raw meat to be good for fertility. First, we shouldn't automatically assume that because something is true in cats, that it will also prove true for humans. We have very different digestive systems. Then with our next story, which does involve human subjects, it is really nothing more than hearsay evidence. Certainly interesting though. I can't prove or disprove its validity. However, I strongly, strongly advise pregnant women not to consume any raw meat! It can pose a serious risk not only to them, but also to their unborn children.

Cooking does remove some of the wonderful nutrients from our foods. Here is a list of the common meat cooking methods and a brief description of their effects on the meat itself...

Grilling: Any of the charred part you are consuming, is said to be a carcinogen. Yes, I'd like my steak well-done sprinkled with a dash of cancer crust, please. Grilling also destroys a good amount of the vitamins and minerals naturally present in your meat.

Frying: I don't think there's any question over how healthy this method is. Since the meat is cooked in its own fat, you'll be really enjoying the taste of those fats and sodium content. This partially explains what makes fried foods so delicious. There's another "yum factor" danger. What are you cooking your meat in? I'm guessing it's probably some form of butter and oil. That likely will not be good news for your arteries. Frying your meat has a whole host of dangers. Its fine in moderation, but a lifestyle of fried foods is going to land you in a heap of trouble.

Boiling: Not as bad as the other methods, but still not great. You will be boiling out the good and bad fats simultaneously.

Microwaving: A great way to kill the living properties of your food, while potentially keeping the germs alive.

Baking: While a better alternative preferable to most of these other methods; baking still kills a lot of the important nutrients within your meat.

Raw Fish

We often hear the two words "sushi" and "sashimi" used interchangeably. However, they are not one in the same. Sushi actually refers to the sticky rice that is cold, cooked, and soaked in vinegar. Sushi may or may not contain raw fish. California (cucumber, avocado, and cooked imitation crab meat) or Kappa Maki (cucumber) Rolls may be up your alley if you're not quite ready, or simply just not interested in, raw fish. Sashimi, on the other hand, is the actual raw fish itself (or any form of raw meat).

Many people may be afraid of sashimi, but oft without due justification. The fish that is captured for eating raw is of a rather high quality. Sashimi is generally safer than raw meat since it is usually specifically sold for raw consumption. The fish tends to come from salt water, which lessens the probability of parasites compared to fish that have been exposed to freshwater somewhere in their lifecycle. Freshwater fish, such as unagi, are not off limits, but they must have been frozen at deep temperatures to eliminate any unnecessary risk. You should never take it upon yourself to capture and eat a raw freshwater fish (or any fish really). Freshwater is a playground for breeding parasites. Salt water mitigates the risks, while fish farms probably present the lowest risk level of all. Nearly half of the fish intended for consumption today have been raised in fish farms.

Freezing

All sashimi fish must be frozen after capture according to FDA regulation, with the exception of tuna. There are many industrial freezers out there that store fish at a bone chilling temperature of NEGATIVE seventy-five degrees Fahrenheit. Flash freezing is a method used by my many professionals to freeze food very quickly at an ultra-low temperature. It is an effective method of eliminating parasites such as Anasakis.

Cross-Contamination

While hearing the word parasite can cause some concern, I wouldn't let that discourage you from enjoying a refreshing plate of sashimi. Cross-contamination is actually a more justified fear than anything being intrinsically wrong with the fish itself. Cross-contamination occurs when the bacteria from one food item transfers to another. This usually takes place with dirty cutting boards, previously used knives, or unwashed hands. For these very reasons, you want to make sure you trust that the restaurant in which you are enjoying your sashimi upholds strict standards of cleanliness.

Mercury

Another concern I often hear in terms of fish consumption is the fear of mercury. This is a realistic concern, but not one that is sufficient enough to deter you from enjoying your favorite toro. A certain amount of mercury is present is all sorts of fish. Unless you are enjoying a diet absent of seafood, there's really no way to avoid it. In fact, consistently enjoying canned tuna is likely more dangerous than sashimi. The reason it's such a source of anxiety in the case of sashimi, is because the fish that is typically selected for raw consumption is of a larger stature. They are predatorial in nature and have therefore consumed a number of fish themselves. Their prey may have also been contaminated with mercury, contributing to their total mercury content. If you're pregnant, you should probably avoid sashimi altogether, since mercury has been linked to certain birth defects.

Sashimi with a lower risk level of mercury include, but are not limited to.... Sandfish (Hatahata), Scallops (Hotategai), Octopus (Tako), Salmon (Sake), Trout (Masu), Crab (Kani), and Squid (Ika).

Sashimi with a higher risk level of mercury include, but are not limited to... Swordfish (Kajiki), Blue Marlin (Makjiki), Mackerel (Saba), Sea Bass (Suzuki), and Albacore Tune (Shiro).

Pollution

Pollution is another worry of sashimi lovers. Polychlorinated biphenyls (PCBs) are one thing in particular. In 1977, the EPA prohibited their production but tons were emitted into the environment prior to then. While we're not seeing these toxins being released today, they do not easily dissolve in water so they are still harming our fish. Other elements of pollution found in the water are oil, trash, pesticides, and sewage. Personally, I find contamination to be something that we unfortunately have deal with in so many facets of life. Sure, we can put safety measures into affect to prevent further harm, but we can't live in a bubble to avoid what's already out there. Pollution is everywhere. It's in the air we breathe, so it should be no surprise that it's found in the oceans and food we eat. It's an unfortunate reality. The reason sashimi is such a concern in particular is because toxins often accumulate in fatty deposits. The fish that are used for sashimi are typically high in fat content and are predatorial in nature so they may carry an unusually high amount of toxins.

Grading Scale

You may be feeling pretty secure when consuming sashimi grade fish and reasonably so. Just don't be confused into believing that it means more than it actually does. I always assumed it meant that the fish had undergone some sort of inspection, were subjected to rigorous standards, and were required to be handled in some particular manner. Turns out, this whole grading scale is only slightly more meaningful than a marketing buzzword. It is an industry term to let chefs know that a particular piece of meat is suitable for raw consumption. The term is not defined, nor policed, by any accountable agency of inspection. Sorry to disappoint you, but there are no sashimi sergeants that poke and prod the sushi distinguishing subtle attributes. There is no sashimi aficionado school. (That I know of at least.) Now don't get me wrong, there are some incredible fish markets where industry experts are able to make some impeccable distinctions amongst various grades of cuts. Yes, there are people out there who know and sort fish based on its quality. I'm just saying that in general, you shouldn't put too much confidence in a label meaning something more than the fish being of an acceptable quality to be consumed raw.

Sashimi Benefits

In reality the chance that you are going to be harmed in any way by your sashimi is rather minuscule. Fortunately cases of sashimi related illnesses are few and far between. Enjoy sashimi from a source you trust to not have incurred cross-contamination. Once again resort to that common sense factor. If you have any reason to believe the establishment serving your sashimi should not be completely trusted, do not eat there. Trust your instincts. Unlike the risks though, the benefits of sashimi consumption are guaranteed.

Omega-3 Fatty Acids - These essential healthy fats found in sashimi are a nutrition underdog. Omega-3s don't quite get the attention they well deserve and I suspect that this will soon change. It's something that our body needs, but is incapable of producing on its own. Omega-3 has been shown to boost our good cholesterol, while lowering the bad. A big problem that is overlooked in our modern diets is that we are not enjoying enough of the good fats. Omega-3s are beneficial for vascular health, blood sugar levels, and the nervous system. A study published by the *Journal of Neuroscience* indicated that there is evidence to show that this fatty acid can even help ward off Alzheimer's Disease. As a rule of thumb, deep cold water residing fish have even higher levels of Omega-3. I began taking fish oil pills with Omega-3s for vanity purposes. It was suggested to me by my stylist to help grow out my hair. I thought it was silly, but figured what did I have to lose besides the heinous mullet from the top of my head. Desperate for a solution to grow out my hair quickly I decided to give these omega-3 fish pills a try. I could not believe how much of a difference they made. I didn't necessarily notice my hair growing quicker but my skin felt so good. Even in the dead of winter and I never suffered from chapped lips so long as I took my fish oil pill on a daily basis.

Protein – Sashimi is high in protein while low in fat. Besides, the fat that is in sashimi is the good kind (see above). Protein is a major concern of those who are on a highly raw diet. They run the risk of becoming deficient since they are not eating a lot of animal products. That is one reason to consider still eating fish as a pescatarian even while avoiding other types of animal flesh.

Vitamin B6 – Sashimi is one of the few sources of this vital nutrient. Vitamin B6 can regulate your moods and circadian rhythm. If that's not enough to convince you it's a good thing, it also does wonders for your skin, eyes, and hair.

Retinol – The retinol found in sashimi is a form of vitamin A that helps aid vision (by helping your eyes adjust from dark to light and vice versa), cell regeneration, and immunity.

Vitamin E - Vitamin E helps prevent cellular damage and eliminate the free radicals floating around your body.

Niacin - Sashimi is a very good source of niacin. Niacin can help improve your circulation, regulate your mood, and lower your LDL cholesterol level.

Nori – If you enjoy raw fish, you have probably tried some nori as the green stuff on the outside of your sushi roll. Nori is extremely nutritious. Due to its oceanic roots, it's no surprise that it contains iodine. Iodine is essential for a healthy thyroid. Just like everything else though, it's all about moderation. Too much iodine can be dangerous, but luckily a clinical study published in *The Journal of Agricultural and Food Chemistry* found that the amounts of nori that we enjoy in a regular serving are not something we should be all too concerned about. Nori is also a HUGE source of vitamin B12! Children should be cautious though as nori can actually have an inverse effect, and cause their B12 levels to drop.

Final Words

When eating raw meat you should exercise extreme caution and proceed at your own risk. Current meat processing methods are often unsanitary and livestock are raised under such oppressive and despicably grotesque conditions. If you want to eat a little meat, enjoy it cooked. At the very least, ensure it has reached a temperature to be considered medium-rare.

Sashimi is a little less risky. The Institute of Medicine released a statement in 2006 stating that for those with a those who are middle-aged, not-pregnant, and with a healthy immune system, the benefits of consuming sashimi outweighs the risks. I very much agree. We take a risk with every single thing we ingest. I'm not going to recommend that you live on a diet solely composed of Big Macs and milkshakes so that you can avoid contracting Anasakis. Maybe overly processed foods don't contain that same risk of foodborne illness, but they will slowly yet surely poison you in other ways.

9 TEN DAYS WORTH OF RAW RECIPES

One of the most common misconceptions about going raw is that you have to eat one plain food at a time. Carrot juice for breakfast. An apple for lunch. A plate of broccoli for dinner. This could not be further from the truth. Here is a ten day meal plan worth of raw vegan recipes to help get you started. You don't have to eat these recipes consecutively or in any particular fashion. Skip around and try that which interests you. You certainly don't want to immediately transition from eating a cooked carnivorous diet to eating a 100% raw vegan diet. Any rapid changes, however beneficial to your health, should be slowly transitioned.

Many of these recipes require long dehydrating times. Plan your recipes at least a day in advance so that you will have adequate time to make any necessary preparations. *Bon appétit!*

DAY 1

Breakfast

Mega Boost Green Juice
Makes 1 Serving

1 kale leaf
2 apples
3 oz. wheatgrass
1 teaspoon of Spirulina powder

1. Juice kale, apple, and wheatgrass.
2. Pour blended juices into a glass.
3. Add Spirulina powder.
4. Stir.
5. Drink immediately. Do not let sit as this beverage will separate.

Lunch

Mediterranean Zucchini Pasta
Makes 2 Servings

2 zucchinis, peeled
1 red bell pepper, chopped
15 cherry tomatoes
5 basil leaves
2 steamed sweet potatoes
1 1/2 tbsp balsamic vinegar
2 tablespoons of cold-pressed olive oil
dash of nutritional yeast

1. Rinse sweet potatoes off in cool water. (Peel skin if desired.)
2. Cube sweet potatoes into bite-size pieces.
3. Place 3/4 of an inch of water into your steam pot and set on stove. Burner should be set on high heat.
4. Lay cubed potatoes on the steaming insert and cover for twenty minutes.
5. Puree olive oil and basil leaves in a blender.

6. Shred zucchini with a hand peeler (or spiralize) as your pasta.
7. Toss zucchini with the puree, sweet potatoes, and all remaining ingredients.
8. Sprinkle with nutritional yeast (if desired).

Snack

Raw French Fries with Ketchup
Makes 2 Servings

French Fries:
2 jicama
1/4 cup cold-pressed olive oil
1 teaspoon turmeric
1/2 teaspoon sea salt

Ketchup:
2 tomatoes
5 sun-dried tomatoes
1/2 teaspoon of stevia
1/2 teaspoon lemon zest
1/2 garlic clove
1/2 cup water
dash of sea salt

French Fries:
1. Slice jicama as you would french fries.
2. Place jicama, olive oil, turmeric, and salt in a bowl. Mix well.
3. Let set for twelve minutes so that the jicama can absorb the oil.
4. Drain the liquid and then remove excess oil from the jicama gently by dabbing them with a paper towel.

Ketchup:
Place all ingredients in a food processor and blend until achieving desired consistency.

** You can even bottle up your leftover ketchup and store it in the refrigerator. Hint, Hint: You may even want to try some on your portobello burger tonight for dinner.

Dinner

Portobello Mushroom Burgers
Makes 2 Servings

4 baby portobello mushroom caps, chopped
2 tablespoon coconut aminos
1 teaspoon liquid smoke
1/2 tablespoon raw agave nectar
1 tablespoon apple cider vinegar
1 cup sunflower seeds
1/4 cup carrot, finely chopped
1/4 cup celery, finely chopped
1/4 cup onions, finely chopped
1/4 cup garlic, finely chopped
1/2 teaspoon thyme

1. Stir coconut aminos, liquid smoke, agave nectar, and apple cider vinegar in a large bowl. This will be your marinade.
2. Add mushrooms and mix well into marinade. Cover and let soak for approximately two hours.
3. In a food processor, grind sunflower seeds until smooth.
4. Remove mushrooms from marinade and place them into a food processor along with the sunflower seeds. Process the mixture until it is smooth but not runny.
5. Add carrot, celery, and thyme into food processor. Turn the processor on and off in pulses until mixture is well-blended.
6. Mold two patties and dehydrate at 110 degrees for approximately 1 hour and 25 minutes. Then flip, and dehydrate for 3 additional hours. (Keep in mind, your patties will shrink as they dehydrate.)
7. Serve your burgers plain, on raw bread, in a wrap, or over some veggies. You can even serve them using lettuce as the bun, with some sliced tomato and cucumbers, if you prefer.

Dessert

Easy Chocolate Guacamole Pudding
Makes 2 Servings

1 large ripened avocado, pitted
1/2 ripened banana, sliced
5 dates, soaked
1 tablespoon of yacon syrup
1/2 teaspoon vanilla extract
2 tablespoons cocoa
1 tablespoon carob powder
1/2 cup water
2 sprigs of mint

1. Mix all ingredients together in a food processor until the consistency is soft and creamy, resembling pudding.
2. Distribute pudding into two serving bowls.
3. Garnish with mint.

DAY 2

Breakfast

Scrumptious Craisenberry Granola
Makes 2 Servings

3/4 cup soaked buckwheat
3 teaspoons ground flaxseed
1/2 cup sunflower seeds
1/2 cup pumpkin seeds
1/2 cup raisins
1/2 cup dried, diced apple
1/3 cup agave nectar
1 tablespoons coconut oil
2 tablespoons water
1 tablespoon cinnamon
dash of nutmeg
dash of sea salt

For Topping:
Organic Blueberries
Organic Raspberries
Sliced Banana

1. Whisk agave nectar, coconut oil, water, salt, nutmeg, and cinnamon together in a bowl.
2. Add in remaining ingredients and coat well.
3. Dehydrate at 120 degrees Fahrenheit for ten hours.

Lunch

Tangy Ranch Salad
Makes 2 Servings

Ranch Flavored Vinaigrette Dressing:
1 cup cashews
1/2 cup water
2 tablespoons lemon juice
2 tablespoons apple cider vinegar
1/2 cup cold-pressed olive oil
2 tablespoons raw honey
2 garlic cloves
2 tablespoons onion powder
1 teaspoon dill
dash of sea salt

Throw all ingredients into a blender and mix at high speed.

Salad:
3 cups of leaves of your choice (Kale, Spinach, Iceberg, etc.)
2 radishes, sliced
1 carrot, grated
1/2 cup of cheddar cheese, grated (substitute with nutritional yeast if desired)
6 baby tomatoes
1/2 cup apple, chopped
1/2 cup cucumber, chopped

Simply toss all ingredients together with Ranch Flavored Vinaigrette Dressing.

Snack

Sweet Potato Chips
Makes 1 Serving

1 sweet potato, peeled
1 teaspoon cold-pressed olive oil
1/2 teaspoon sea salt

1. Thinly slice sweet potato.
2. Coat in salt and olive oil.
3. Dehydrate until achieving desired consistency.

Dinner

Carrot Falafel Accented with Savory Tahini
Makes 2 Servings

Falafels:
2 1/2 cups carrot pulp (leftover from juicing)
1 cup sesame seeds, ground
3 teaspoons flax seed, ground
2 teaspoons lemon juice
3 tablespoons hemp oil
1 stalk celery, finely chopped
1/2 cup parsley, finely chopped
1/2 cup basil, finely chopped
1 teaspoon cumin
1 clove garlic, finely minced
1/3 cup onion, finely minced
dash of sea salt

Savory Tahini Dressing:
3 teaspoons sesame seeds
1 teaspoon sesame oil
1/3 cup water
3 cloves garlic, crushed
2 tablespoons cold-pressed olive oil

1/4 cup lemon juice
1 teaspoon parsley, finely chopped
dash of sea salt

Falafels:
1. Mix all ingredients together by hand in a large bowl.
2. Roll your falafel into balls, as if you were making meatballs.
3. Flatten slightly using a fork.
4. Dehydrate falafels at 120 degrees for approximately two hours.
5. Flip and repeat.

Savory Tahini:
1. Grind sesame seeds in food processor until smooth.
2. Add in the remaining ingredients and blend well.
3. Drizzle onto falafel for a delicious treat.

Dessert

Unbaked Brownie Delight
Makes Several Servings

2 cups walnuts, whole
3 cups Medjool dates, pitted
1 teaspoon of agave nectar
1 cup raw cacao
1 cup raw unsalted almonds, chopped
1/4 teaspoon sea salt

1. Finely grind walnuts in a food processor on high.
2. Add agave nectar, cacao, and sea salt.
3. Pulse until well mixed.
4. Add dates one at a time into the food processor while running. (The consistency will appear crumby, but will hold together when pressed.)
5. Pour mixture into pan and top with chopped almonds.
6. Freeze mixture in an airtight container for at least one hour.
7. Slice and serve.

DAY 3

Breakfast

Just Peachy Morning Smoothie
Makes 1 Serving

1 ripe frozen peach, chopped and peeled
1/2 cup Greek yogurt
1 tablespoon agave nectar
3 ice cubes

Blend until achieving desired consistency.

Lunch

Refreshing Cucumber Soup
Makes 2 Servings

1 1/2 cucumbers, diced
1/2 cup avocado, chopped
1 garlic clove
2 teaspoons cold-pressed olive oil
1/2 cup water
2 heaping teaspoons sweet onion, chopped
1 tablespoon parsley, finely minced
dash of sea salt
dash of pepper

1. Puree 1 peeled cucumber for thirty seconds. (Leaving the remaining 1/2 for later.)
2. Add olive oil, garlic, parsley, water, and avocado. Puree in blender for a minute and a half.
3. Pour into serving bowls.
4. Add sweet onions, salt, pepper, and remaining cucumber with peel as topping.

Snack

Sprout Salad
Makes 1 Serving

1/4 cup mung bean sprouts
1/2 cup sunflower greens
1/2 cup alfalfa sprouts
1/2 cup buckwheat lettuce, chopped
1/4 cup fenugreek sprouts
cold pressed olive oil (as desired)

Toss all ingredients.

Dinner

Tangy Thai Lettuce Wraps
Makes 2 Servings

1 head of lettuce
1/4 cup celery, diced
1/4 cup carrots, diced
1/3 cup red bell pepper, diced
1/4 cup fresh cilantro, minced
1/4 cup scallion greens, minced
mung bean sprouts (for topping)
grated carrot (for topping)

Dipping Sauce:
1/4 cup agave nectar
1/8 cup Nama Shoyu (or soy sauce)
1/2 teaspoon fresh minced garlic
1 teaspoons fresh grated ginger
1 teaspoon sesame seeds, hulled
1 teaspoon sesame oil
1 teaspoon red pepper flakes
3/4 cup walnuts

1. Pull apart large lettuce leaves. Wash and dry.
2. Place all sauce ingredients, except walnuts, into food processor and pulse three times.
3. Add walnuts to sauce and pulse three times.
4. Add remaining vegetable ingredients from lettuce wraps and pulse 3 times with sauce mixture.
5. Lay out lettuce leaves and place three tablespoons of the mixture onto the leaf.
6. Garnish with mung sprouts and grated carrots.

Dessert

Carrot Cake Cupcakes with Cream Cheese Frosting
Makes 4 Servings

Carrot Cake:
1/2 cup walnuts
1/2 cup dates
1 cup carrot pulp (from juicing)
1/2 teaspoon cinnamon
1/4 teaspoon ginger
1/8 teaspoon sea salt
1/4 cup raisins
1/4 cup dried apricots
dash of nutmeg

Cream Cheese Frosting:
1/2 cup cashews, soaked
3 dates, pitted and soaked
1/2 teaspoon lemon juice
1/2 teaspoon coconut milk
2 drops of stevia
dash of sea salt
shredded coconut (for topping)

Cake:
1. Blend dates and walnuts in a food processor for thirty seconds.
2. Add spices and carrot pulp, blending until dough-like.
3. Add raisins and apricots and pulse two times.

4. Pour batter into cupcake molds.
5. Refrigerate for 1 1/2 hours.

Frosting:
1. Add all frosting ingredients into food processor and blend to desired consistency.
2. After the cakes have been refrigerated sufficiently apply frosting.
3. Top with shredded coconut.

DAY 4

Breakfast

Energizing Oatmeal
Makes 1 Serving

1 apple, chopped
1/2 banana, sliced
1/2 tablespoon golden flaxseed, soaked
1 teaspoon cinnamon
1/3 cup of almond cream
1 teaspoon of hemp seeds

1. Rinse soaked flaxseeds.
2. Place all ingredients into blender. Blend until smooth.

Lunch

Squash Spaghetti Coated in a Classic Italian Tomato Sauce
Makes 2 Servings

2 yellow summer squash
3 tomatoes
3 sun-dried tomatoes
1 garlic clove
2 basil leaves
1 teaspoon oregano
1/2 tablespoon pepper, freshly ground
1/4 cup onions, chopped

1/4 cup cold-pressed olive oil
2 tablespoons lemon juice
2 dates, pitted
2 olives, pitted
dash of sea salt

1. Spiralize squash.
2. Sprinkle squash with a drizzle of olive oil and a dash of salt.
3. Let sit for five minutes.
4. Place remaining ingredients in blender and blend at high speed until creamy.
5. Plate spaghetti and pour sauce over dish.

Snack

Midday Hummus
Makes 1 Serving

1 cup garbanzo beans, sprouted
1/2 cup cold-pressed olive oil
1/4 cup raw tahini
2 garlic cloves
2 tablespoons lime juice, fresh squeezed
dash of sea salt

Blend ingredients together until achieving a creamy consistency. Use as a dip for your favorite fruits and vegetables.

Dinner

Quick Cabbage Salad
Makes 2 Servings (with leftovers)

1 head cabbage, shredded
2 carrots, shredded
2 avocados, pitted
1 lemon, juiced
2 tablespoons whole grain mustard

1. Mix cabbage and carrot together in a large bowl.

2. Blend remaining ingredients until smooth.
3. Pour sauce over vegetables and toss well.

Dessert

Healthy Oatmeal Cookies
Makes Several Servings

1 banana, ripened
1 tablespoon maple syrup
1 teaspoon cold-pressed olive oil
1 cup oats
1 tablespoon flax seed
1/2 tablespoon cinnamon
1/3 teaspoon cardamom, ground
2 dates, pitted and chopped
1 tablespoon raisins
1 teaspoon ginger, finely diced
2 walnuts, crushed

1. Mash banana in a large bowl.
2. Add in olive oil and maple syrup.
3. Slowly add remaining ingredients, mixing as you combine.
4. Scoop 1-inch balls of your mixture onto a lined tray and dehydrate at 110 degrees for one whole day (or as desired).

DAY 5

Breakfast

Scrumptious Groats and Oats
Makes 1 Serving

1 ½ cups oat groats, soaked
1/3 cup dates, pitted
1/3 cup raisins
1/4 teaspoon cinnamon
2 teaspoons water

Mix all of the ingredients together in a food processor until achieving desired consistency.

Lunch

Mediterranean Pizza
Makes 2 Servings

Pizza Crust:
1 cup rutabaga, cubed
1 cup jicama, cubed
1/4 cup zucchini, peeled cubed
2 1/4 cups walnuts, soaked
1/3 cup flax seeds, ground
1/4 cups hemp seeds
1 teaspoon sea salt
2 tablespoons water

Pizza Sauce:
2 cups cashews, soaked
3 teaspoons raw sesame tahini
1 garlic clove
1/3 cup lemon juice
1/2 teaspoon ground cumin
1/3 cup water
1/2 teaspoon sea salt
dash of cayenne pepper

Olive Pate Topping:
1 1/4 cups green olives, finely chopped and pitted
2 teaspoons fresh dill
1 teaspoon freshly squeezed lemon juice
1/3 cup cold-pressed olive oil

Optional Toppings:
Cherry Tomatoes
Green olives
Mushrooms
Red pepper

dash of freshly ground black pepper
dash of sea salt
nutritional yeast (as desired)

Dough:
1. Blend rutabaga, jicama, zucchini, and walnuts in food processor until chopped into small pieces, but not to the extent where they are pureed.
2. Place mixture into a large bowl.
3. Add remaining pizza dough ingredients.
4. Mix by hand.
5. Lay out dough onto a lined round dehydrator tray.
6. Dehydrate at 115 degrees for approximately eight hours.
7. Flip and dehydrate for another two hours.
8. Cut dough into slices once firm.
9. Dehydrate slices for one hour.

Pizza Sauce:
1. Add all ingredients (except for water) into blender.
2. Gradually pour in water until attaining a paste-like consistency.

For Olive Pate Topping: Combine all ingredients in a food processor until well mixed.

Assembly:
1. Lay out pizza dough.
2. Dress with sauce.
3. Add Olive Pate as desired.
4. Affix selected toppings.

Snack

Raw Vegan Bacon
Makes 2 Servings

1 eggplant, thinly sliced lengthwise in strips
1/2 cup cold-pressed olive oil
2 teaspoons apple cider vinegar

2 teaspoons plum vinegar
3 teaspoons maple syrup
2 teaspoons cider
1 teaspoon of liquid smoke
dash of freshly ground pepper

1. Place all ingredients (except for zucchini) into a small bowl and stir well.
2. Line your eggplant strips in a pan.
3. Pour mixture over eggplant.
4. Marinate in refrigerator for two hours.
5. Remove eggplant and dehydrate for ten hours.

Dinner

Cabbage Tacos
Makes 2 Servings

8 red cabbage leaves
2 carrots, shredded
1 cup alfalfa sprouts
1/2 avocado, mashed
2 teaspoons freshly squeezed lemon juice
6 stalks chives, finely chopped
dash of seaweed flakes
dash of sea salt

1. Mash avocado, lemon juice, chives, and sea salt together. Mix well.
2. Utilizing the cabbage as your taco shell, add the avocado mixture as your base.
3. Top with sprouts, carrot, and seaweed flakes.

Dessert

Cherry Banana Ice Cream
Makes 1 Serving

2 frozen bananas, sliced
1/2 teaspoon vanilla extract
Frozen cherries (as desired)

1. Place bananas and vanilla extract into food processor. Blend until creamy.
2. Add cherries and pulse three times.
3. Freeze for two hours.

DAY 6

Breakfast

Raw Porridge
Makes 1 Serving

1 cup raw oat groats, soaked
2 tablespoons almonds
1/4 teaspoon lucuma powder
1/4 teaspoon cinnamon
1 teaspoon honey
1/4 cup water
dash of salt
fresh berries (as desired)

1. Process all ingredients, except berries, into food processor until achieving a smooth consistency.
2. Garnish with berries.

Lunch

Nori Rolls
Makes 2 Rolls

2 nori sheets
1/4 red pepper, julienned
1 avocado, sliced
1/3 cup bean sprouts
1/3 cup alfalfa sprouts

1 tomato, sliced
1 cucumber, julienned
1/2 zucchini, shredded
Sesame Seeds
Nama Shoyu (for dipping)

1. Lay down nori sheets on a flat surface.
2. Moisten the outer two inches with the sliced tomato.
3. Apply a thin layer of each ingredient onto the sushi roll, leaving the outer two edges uncovered.
4. Roll up nori tightly. Slicing the roll into approximately eight pieces.
5. Cover in sesame seeds.
6. Dip in Nama Shoyu.

Snack

Raw Bruschetta
Makes 10 Pieces

Bruschetta:
1 cup golden flaxseeds, ground to mill
3 teaspoons water
4 tablespoons cold-pressed olive oil

Topping:
3 tablespoons cold-pressed olive oil
10 round tomato slices
pinch of dried thyme, ground
pinch of oregano, ground
pinch of basil, ground
pinch of marjoram, ground
pinch of garlic, ground

Bruschetta:
1. Add bruschetta ingredients together and mix well.
2. Mold ten bruschetta crackers.
3. Place crackers in dehydrator for approximately three hours (or until crispy).

Topping:
1. Pour olive oil and seasonings into a bowl. Stir well.
2. Add tomato slices to marinade and let sit for the three hours (while bruschetta crackers dehydrate).

Assemble by placing a slice of tomato over your cracker and drizzling olive oil on top.

Dinner

Hearty Raw Soup
Makes 1 Serving

2 tomatoes, ripened and chopped
1/2 red apple, chopped
¼ red bell pepper, chopped
1/3 cucumber, chopped
1/2 avocado, chopped
1/2 green onion, chopped
1/2 teaspoon pumpkin seeds, ground
2 tablespoons cold-pressed olive oil
1 garlic clove
dash of sea salt
dash of seaweed flakes
dash of fresh pepper
dash of basil

Blend all ingredients together until obtaining desired consistency.

Dessert

Spicy Spanish Sesame Brownies
Makes Several Servings

1/3 cup sesame seeds, hulled and ground
1/4 cup cacao powder
4 teaspoons agave nectar
2 teaspoons cold-pressed coconut oil

1/2 teaspoon cinammon
1/2 teaspoon cardamon
1/4 teaspoon cayenne

1. Mix all ingredients together in a large bowl.
2. Transfer mixture into a pan.
3. Refrigerate for one hour.

DAY 7

Breakfast

Morning Mush
Makes 1 Serving

1 sweet potato, peeled and chopped
7 dates, seedless
1/2 cup coconut milk
1 banana, sliced
dash of nutmeg
dash of cinnamon

1. Add all ingredients, except for banana, into food processor. Blend until creamy.
2. Scoop your mixture into two bowls and garnish with banana slices.

Lunch

Pad Thai
Makes 1 Serving

3/4 cup raw cashews, soaked
4 teaspoons raw honey
2 tablespoons Bragg's Liquid Aminos
2 teaspoons apple cider vinegar
3 strips of dried kelp, chopped
1 cup bean sprouts
5 snap peas

1. Blend cashews until smooth.
2. Add honey, liquid aminos, and apple cider vinegar to blended cashews and mix well.
3. Lay a bed of your bean sprouts across a plate.
4. Layer kelp a top of the sprouts.
5. Pour your cashew sauce on top.
6. Garnish with snap peas.

Snack

Cream of Spinach Soup
Makes 1 Serving

1½ cup spinach
2 cups water
1/2 teaspoon cold-pressed olive oil
1/2 zucchini, peeled
1/2 tomato
1/4 cup hemp seeds
1/4 cup sunflower seeds
1/2 teaspoon garlic cloves, diced
1/2 teaspoon sea salt
1 teaspoon onion, diced
1 teaspoon cumin
1/2 teaspoon of curry powder
dash of pepper, freshly ground

1. Blend spinach, water, olive oil, and seeds until smooth.
2. Add all remaining ingredients and blend until mixture obtains a soup-like consistency.

Dinner

Vegetable Lo Mein
Makes 2 Servings

1 1/4 tablespoons Nama Shoya
1 1/4 tablespoons apple cider vinegar
1 tablespoon raw agave nectar

2 teaspoon sesame oil
1/4 teaspoon powdered ginger
1 zucchini, spiralized
1 carrot, spiralized
1/2 cup sliced mushrooms
1/2 cup sugar snap peas in pod, whole
1/4 cup bean sprouts

1. Toss all ingredients together in a large bowl.
2. Let sit for twenty minutes.
3. Toss once more prior to serving.

Dessert

Cheese-less Pineapple Cheesecake
Makes Several Servings

1 peeled apple, chopped
3/4 cup cashews, soaked
9 dates, pitted
1/2 cup flaxseed, ground
1/2 cup orange juice
1/2 lemon, fresh squeezed juice
1 tablespoon coconut oil
2 cups pineapple, diced
dash of salt
sprinkle of orange rind
kiwi slices for garnish

1. Blend all ingredients in food processor, except for pineapple and kiwi.
2. Pour contents into bottom of pan as crust.
3. Blend pineapple and pour on top of cashew crust.
4. Garnish with sliced kiwis and orange rind.

DAY 8

Breakfast

Green Gas: Body Fuel
Makes 1 Serving

1/2 cup spinach
3 stalks celery
1/3 cucumber, with skin
1/2 apple

1. Rinse and juice all ingredients, one at a time
2. Drink immediately.

Lunch

All Alkaline Salad
Makes 1 Serving

1 cup romaine
1/2 avocado, sliced
1/2 apple, chopped
1/2 cucumber, chopped
5 baby carrots
2 teaspoons of raisins
1/2 cup alfalfa sprouts
3 teaspoons cold-pressed olive oil
2 teaspoons apple cider vinegar

Toss all of the ingredients well in a large bowl and that's all there is to it. (You can replace the olive oil and vinegar with your choice of dressing as desired.)

Snack

Miso Soup
Makes 2 Servings

2 tablespoons organic brown rice miso

1 ½ tablespoons coconut oil
2 cups hot water (temperature as desired for soup)
1 teaspoon Nori flakes
8 Brazil nuts

1. Add coconut oil, water, and Nori flakes into blender for twenty seconds.
2. Let sit for thirty seconds.
3. Add remaining ingredients and blend until achieving desired consistency.

Dinner

Lentil Spout Avocado Bowls
Makes 2 Servings

1 ½ cups celery, minced
1 teaspoon raw sesame tahini
5 cups lentils, sprouted
1/4 cup raw almond butter
1/2 cup water
1/4 cup cold-pressed olive oil
4 teaspoons Bragg's Aminos
1 red pepper, chopped
1 green onions with tops, minced
1 teaspoon kelp
4 avocados, halved and pitted

** When sprouting your lentils, it will take approximately 3 cups to furnish 5 cups worth of sprouts. The sprouting process should take around 48 hours in total. Be sure to rinse your sprouts at least twice daily.

1. Blend almond butter, olive oil, and water in blender until smooth.
2. Blend lentil sprouts in food processor and then pour into large bowl.
3. Mix in remaining ingredients and almond butter mixture.
4. Stir well and refrigerate for five hours.

5. When ready to serve add the mixture into the center of the avocados.

Dessert

Berry Sorbet
Makes 2 Servings

1 cup vanilla Greek yogurt
1/2 cup blueberries
1/2 cup mango
1/2 cup strawberries

1. Blend until well mixed.
2. Pour mixture into a sealed container and chill in freezer for a minimum of thirty minutes.

DAY 9

Breakfast

Coconut Cake Bars
Makes 2 Servings

1 tablespoon coconut oil
2 cups flax meal
3 tablespoons raw agave nectar
¼ teaspoon sea salt
1 teaspoon of shredded coconut

1. Toss all ingredients into a large bowl and stir well.
2. Once mixture is well blended, roll out the batter on a flat surface.
3. Slice into desired size servings.
4. Dehydrate. (Optional)

Lunch

Raw Mac and Cheese
Makes 1 Serving

2 zucchinis, shredded
1/3 cup red pepper, shredded
2 tablespoons water
2 teaspoons cold-pressed olive oil
2 teaspoons nutritional yeast
dash of garlic powder
dash of onion power
dash of sea salt
crushed walnuts (as desired)

1. Place shredded zucchini into a large bowl.
2. Blend remaining ingredients (minus the walnuts).
3. Pour mixture over noodles and stir.
4. Dehydrate for 1 ½ hours.
5. Sprinkle walnuts on top and serve.

Snack

Cabble Salad
Makes 2 Servings

2 cups red cabbage, shredded
1 golden delicious apple, chopped
2 teaspoons raisins
1/4 cup walnuts
1/3 cup apple cider vinegar
2 tablespoons cold-pressed olive oil
2 tablespoons honey
dash of salt
dash of black pepper

Toss all ingredients in a bowl until well mixed.

Dinner

Collard Green Tacos
Makes 2 Servings

1/3 cup nuts of choice, soaked
1/2 cup sunflower seeds, soaked
1/3 cup almonds, soaked
1/3 cup water
2 stalks celery
2 tablespoons lemon juice, fresh squeezed
2 teaspoons cold-pressed olive oil
1 teaspoon raw agave nectar
1 tomato, chopped
10 collard greens

1. Blend together all ingredients, except collard greens and tomatoes, in a food processor.
2. Scoop mixture onto collard green leaves along with a spoonful of tomato.

Dessert

Chocolate Coconut Mousse
Makes 1 Serving

1 coconut
2 tablespoons cacao powder
3 ice cubes

Place coconut water and meat into blender along with remaining ingredients. Blend until creamy.

DAY 10

Breakfast

Chocolate Cereal
Makes 1 Serving

1/2 cup wheat, soaked
1/3 cup almonds, soaked
1/3 cup raisins
1 tablespoon raw cacao powder
1 teaspoon raw agave nectar

Mix all ingredients together and enjoy.

Lunch

Sprout Salad
Makes 1 Serving

1/2 cucumber, chopped
1/2 apple, chopped
1/2 zucchini, chopped
1/2 cup wheat berry sprouts
1/2 cup alfalfa sprouts
1/3 avocado, chopped
1/2 cup edamame beans
1/4 cup cold-pressed olive oil

Toss all ingredients together and serve.

Snack

Sweet and Savory Snack Dip
Makes 1 Serving

2 tablespoons raw honey
1 tablespoon raw tahini

1 apple sliced
10 baby carrots

1. Stir honey and tahini mixture.
2. Dip apple slices and carrots into savory dip.

Dinner

Delectable Dinner Wraps
Makes 1 Serving

4 large iceberg lettuce leaves
2 tomatoes, chopped
3 garlic cloves, minced
1 cup corn, kernels
1 teaspoon lime juice, fresh squeezed
1/4 cup cilantro, chopped
1 teaspoon onion, chopped

1. Place avocado in a large bowl and mash.
2. Add remaining ingredients (except for lettuce leaves). Stir well.
3. Add two teaspoons of mixture onto each lettuce leaf.

Dessert

Coconut Snowball Cookies
Makes Several Servings

2 cups almonds
1 1/2 cups raisins
1 cup dried coconut, shredded

1. Blend almonds and raisins in food processor until achieving a dough-like consistency.
2. Mold the dough into balls.
3. Roll in coconut.
4. Refrigerate for one hour.

10 TEN TAKEAWAYS FOR SUCCESS

With the myriad of nutrition experts and diet plans out there we can become overwhelmed. Whether for better health, vanity, or nutrition stop dieting and just start eating right. Use these ten quick and simple rules to change your lifestyle for the better.

#10 Eat More Fruits & Vegetables - It's as easy as keeping them in the house. You can only eat what's in front of you. Stop stocking your pantry and start furnishing your fridge. Usually diets fail because people eat too much bad food, not because they didn't eat enough good food. The more you fill up on that which your body needs, the less room you'll have for the junk.

#9 Opt For Organic Whenever Possible - "Organic" is not a meaningless buzzword. By eating clean you will stay in the clear from all sorts of poisons and your food will be packed with a higher concentration of vitamins and nutrients. It may not be the most frugal way to shop for produce, but incredibly worth your while.

#8 Cut Out Processed Foods From Your Diet By A Minimum of 80% - Expecting to stay away from processed foods altogether is pretty much impossible in this day and age. And frankly it's unrealistic to expect that we can always find something fresh on the go. You're not going to stumble across an acai berry smoothie in a vending machine or at a drive through. Just say no to restaurant foods and anything from a box and/or wrapped in plastic whenever possible.

#7 Eat More Alkaline Foods – Disease thrives in acidity. Don't give illness a chance to flourish. A diet rich in raw fruits and vegetables is naturally alkaline, so this step should be a breeze.

#6 Drink At Least 2 Juices Per Day - Replace your sweet calorie loaded beverages in a day (such as coffee and soda) with fresh juices. It would be nearly impossible for most of us to eat the recommended daily servings of fruits and vegetables without the aid of a juicer.

#5 Never Touch Anything Containing Aspartame - Unless you are a masochist or suicidal, then in that case, it might be right up your alley.

#4 Don't Cut Out Your Favorite Foods, Eat Them In Moderation - Stop dieting. Emphasize making it a priority to integrate more good foods into your diet rather than subtracting the bad ones. When you say you're never going to eat your guilty pleasures ever again, you are deceiving yourself. Be honest about your goals and expectations.

#3 Ensure You Are Meeting Your Basic Nutritional Requirements – This is especially a concern for those who are going nearly 100% raw and/or vegan. Take a supplement and ensure that your diet is as varied as possible.

#2 Keep Your Meals Interesting - Be open to new foods and recipes. When you stop eating out of a box, you have all the power in the world to customize your meals in innovative and exciting ways.

#1 GO RAW - You don't have to go 100%, nor should you. Just remember, raw food is real food. By following takeaway #6, 50% of your diet will become raw effortlessly. When you fuel your body with the enzymes, vitamins, and nutrients it needs you immediately begin to restore youth, health, and vitality naturally.

"Let food be thy medicine, and let thy medicine be food."
- Hippocrates

"All that man needs for health and healing has been provided by God in nature, the challenge of science is to find it."
- Philippus Theophrastrus of Aureolus Paracelsus

"The doctor of the future will no longer treat the human frame with drugs, but rather will cure and prevent disease with nutrition."
- Thomas Edison

ESSENTIALLY RAW

ABOUT THE AUTHOR

Marie Sarantakis is a graduate of Carthage College, where she studied political science, philosophy, and the sociology of religion as a Clausen Scholar. In 2010, she was a Wingspread Fellow of the Johnson Foundation and in 2007 recognized with a Patterson Leadership Award. She has presented her research before the Wisconsin Institute for Peace & Conflict Resolution Studies, Society for the Scientific Study of Religion, and American Sociological Association. Miss Sarantakis is currently pursuing her Juris Doctorate from The John Marshall Law School of Chicago, Illinois. She is fluent in Greek and enjoys to travel abroad. In 2009 she was named the 16th Sexiest International Model by Nifty Magazine. Miss Sarantakis continues to enjoy modeling and promoting nutrition to audiences worldwide.

Made in the USA
Lexington, KY
11 February 2013